COCO BERLIN

Pussy Yoga

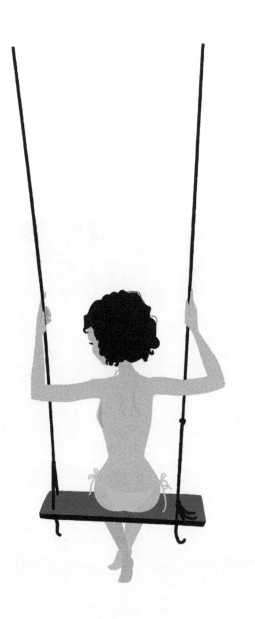

COCO BERLIN

Pussy Yoga

Pelvic Floor Training for Radiance,
Confidence, and a Fulfilling Love Life

Translation: Rebecca Darby, Anne Kavanagh

Editing: Kat Pedersen, Anne Kavanagh

Proof: Will Tyler

Illustration: Keike Kmiotek

Design: Lydia Kühn, Anton Khodakovsky

ISBN   978-84-09-28560-0   hardcover
        978-84-09-28594-5   e-book

Contents

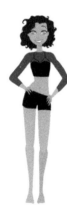

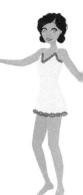

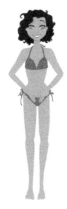

Sensuality and Sex

Preface

To my great delight, my belly dance teacher of many years has written this wonderful book, *Pussy Yoga*. Some might find the title provocative, but I love it! It brings to mind the image of a cat lying in the sun, relaxed and content. Then she gets up, stretches and lengthens her body, and then centered in herself, she moves with elegance, using muscles that are strong but not rigid. Few women today move in such a supple way, and it's a joy to watch those who can. The way we live and treat our bodies divorces us from our sensuousness and self-awareness.

The pelvic floor is the control center of the female body, but many women know little about it. As a gynecologist, I ask my patients to engage their pelvic floors every day. Most of them jerk their pelvis forward, clench their glutes tightly, and suck in their lower abdominal muscles, forcing their bladder downward. Their pelvic floor doesn't change state. It's either not involved in the movement at all, or it's much too tight. The pelvis and all of its muscles aren't only important for preventing incontinence and back pain; a strong upright posture also has its root in the pelvic floor. In fact, the muscle tone of the pelvic floor and the position of the pelvis reveal a lot about the way a woman faces life in general.

The pelvic floor is the seat of our passion, our pleasure, and our lust—with or without a partner. It's high time we started treating our pussy in a positive, joyous, and relaxed way.

I hope you enjoy your journey!

Kiel, Germany, April 2018
Dorothee Struck, M.D., PhD,
Gynecologist & Obstetrician

What You Can Expect from This Book

Welcome to the discovery of your sensuous power. This book will help you get friendly with your pussy, your pelvic floor, and your amazing body. It will help you rediscover yourself from the inside and tap into your own hidden potential.

Since I first experienced the power of sensuous pelvic floor training for myself, and then saw how this knowledge and technique liberated my students, I've been on a mission to share this information with as many women as possible. I want to help every woman realize that she is the source of her own power.

> Not only a fulfilling love life, but everything you long for is already inside of you. You'll find the key to unlock it in this book.

Women who are sensuously aware of their pelvic floor and know how to use it are authentic, powerful, and sexy. They're aligned with themselves. They know what they want, and they have the mental clarity and physical energy to achieve whatever they desire.

They express their sexuality with passion and enjoy life to the fullest. They sparkle with vitality and maintain that fresh radiance their entire lives. Through satisfying sex, orgasms, and the resulting emotional intimacy, these women hold the essential elements for fulfilling and intimate romantic relationships in the palm of their hands.

This inner power is available to every woman, and you will begin to feel it after your first few Pussy Yoga practices.

The latest scientific research shows that orgasms and a satisfying love life make women feel more sure of themselves, more creative, and more courageous. But a supple pelvis and a properly trained pelvic floor don't just make wonderful orgasms possible; they also create a confident, strong posture, they boost our mental well-being, and they help foster a deeper connection with ourselves.

Sensuous awareness of the body is the only way to find and train the pelvic floor effectively. But cultivating that awareness also creates a stronger connection between mind and body, enhancing physical and mental vitality. Everything you learn in this book is part of a self-reinforcing cycle that, once set in motion, builds on itself in more and more positive ways.

And the best part is this: everything you need is already inside your own wonderful body. You can look forward to an intuitive and, for most women, deeply moving and surprising journey—a journey to yourself. A journey to the lost wisdom of your body. But don't worry, this book does not contain any rote training that demands that you push yourself to succeed. This book is more like a spa visit to yourself, from which you emerge into life feeling sensuous, relaxed, and full of energy.

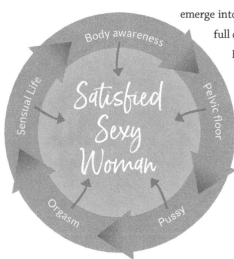

First and foremost, it's about enjoying yourself. All you need is five minutes a day and two or three thirty-minute Pussy Yoga sessions per week. If you want, you can do more. Many women, myself included, love to start the day with our own personalized sensuous workout.

But you don't have to be rigid about it; just follow your own intuition and flow.

After a few sessions, you'll have internalized enough Pussy Yoga to engage your pelvic floor and your new sensuous body awareness automatically throughout your day. You'll use your personal Pussy Yoga practices as needed to relax and reconnect with yourself. The experience is not only incredibly relaxing but is also full of aha moments that will have a huge impact on your life.

We'll advance in stages, and you'll notice big shifts at every step. But don't stop at the first sign of success. There's still more to come! At first, the changes might feel unfamiliar or maybe even a little threatening. After all, it means leaving your old self-image behind. But new horizons await your newly liberated self on the other side.

The information in this book consists of theory, a large section devoted to the Pussy Yoga practices, and tips to further develop your sensuousness in everyday life. So you can read up on the Pussy Science at your own pace, have fun with the practices, and get some inspiration for a more sensually fulfilling life.

1. A New Body Awareness

Pussy Yoga connects your mind and body through a process of sensuous awareness. Most women have a blind spot when it comes to their pelvis and a lot of confusion about where their pelvic floor is—and you can't train what you can't feel in your body. The sensuous component of the practices combines mindfulness and somatic movement with ideokinesis (the art of using imagery and visualization to improve how the body functions and moves). This approach helps your nervous system forge new connections. You'll free yourself from old, restrictive habits in the way you move and behave, the way you think, and the way you feel—without having to overanalyze anything and instead using the wisdom of your own body. Clearing away old patterns and mental blocks is essential to creating a fulfilling and uninhibited love life. Going forward, you'll not only have more fun in bed, but you'll find yourself generally living more freely, creatively, and with greater ease.

Most people live in a state of unconsciousness: they only know passion from the movies and have no idea what they're missing. But once we switch on our sensuousness, we wake up. We come into our bodies. We have more clarity and are more present: we can finally release our inner hand brake and hit the gas.

Sensuousness is something we women have lost, and on an unconscious level, we are always missing it—the ability to feel deeply, to trust our intuition, to give ourselves over to joy and ecstasy of the moment. It's the reason we often feel empty and insecure, the reason we don't trust life or even ourselves. This emptiness is uncomfortable. We try to change ourselves, try to think more positive thoughts, but deep inside, we can never escape this unease.

And when we can no longer stand the emptiness, we numb our bodies so we don't have to feel it anymore. We distract and soothe ourselves with things like food, exercise, work, media consumption, constant social media check-ins, spiritual study, and so on—all of which are fine on their own and flood our bodies with feel-good hormones in the short term. But when we indulge them compulsively, as a comforting distraction, they become an addiction. They no longer serve us but instead leave us feeling dull and frustrated.

In my experience (and the latest psychological research backs this up), the only solution to this alienation from self lies in mind-body integration, and reclaiming intense, sensuous feeling. In recent years, this

When I had an eating disorder, Coco inspired me to take my first steps toward valuing myself and getting back in touch with my poor, starving body.

Sophie Lotta,
Instagram influencer and author

has proven to be the only tried and true approach known to provide long-term healing to victims of trauma.[1] A stronger connection to your body spawns a new self-image. A new sensuous awareness of our body upgrades our perception of ourselves and immediately boosts our self-confidence.

Genuine self-confidence—confidence that comes from the body—makes life more enjoyable. Unfortunately, it isn't something our culture encourages: after all, women who are dissatisfied with themselves are more reliable consumers and are easier to manipulate.[2] But we can reclaim our power with help from our body. A body-centered approach is not only easier; it's also more sustainable than working with the mind alone.[3]

Sensual awareness brings you into the here and now. The practices in this book will help you to fully arrive in your body. If we're constantly living in our heads (as most women today are), it's hard to allow ourselves to even access our sensuality, never mind fully develop it. If you ignite your sensuality with the help of the practices in this book and then let it blaze all day long, you'll fall in love with your body and with life. You'll feel more confident and have more fun flirting, enjoying sex and amazing orgasms.

That's not to say that you'll be thinking about sex all day—though that can be a side effect in the beginning. But don't worry about turning into a nymphomaniac. You'll soon find your own balance where you can enjoy the beauty of life with all your senses and pursue your goals with inspiration and creativity at the same time.

> Thanks to Coco, I feel relaxed and strong every day and, at the same time, so sexy and feminine. That's priceless to me!
>
> Hannah Mang, copywriter and communications coach

2. The Power of the Pelvic Floor

In a survey of four thousand women ages twenty-five to eighty-four, epidemiologist Jean Lawrence found that one in three women has at least one pelvic floor dysfunction. Her research dispelled the myth that pelvic floor problems only affect older women.[4] In fact, through improper exercises, too much sitting (and too little movement in general), stress, the objectification of our bodies, and society's hostility to pleasure, most women's pelvic floors have atrophied and, in addition, are often quite tight.

In Pussy Yoga, we dive deep into the secret world of the pelvis and get to know the mysterious pelvic floor. Most women think the pelvic floor is only the set of muscles surrounding the pussy, but it's a much larger and more powerful musculofascial network. Ideally, it should be fully integrated with the rest of your body because it is the center of your musculoskeletal system. Its fitness and integration have a direct impact on the overall health and alignment of your entire body.

A loose or tense pelvic floor pulls the pelvic bones out of balance, which in turn leads to poor posture. As a result, internal organs can slide downwards, and important nerves can end up being pinched, which means they can no longer transmit sexy sensations to your brain. An activated pelvic floor stimulates the nerves in your entire pelvic area, making you more sensitive and orgasmic—and making your pussy stronger.

Only when you get to know your pelvic floor in its entirety and activate it dynamically (instead of just tightening it up with the wrong exercises) can you can take advantage of its full power! The pelvic floor is a true marvel. An awakened, relaxed, and well-trained pelvic floor will give you a new zest for life. It will straighten your posture and ground you. Studies have shown that people with a fit pelvic floor are much healthier physically, mentally, and emotionally, and are better able to deal with the demands of life than people who do not train their pelvic floors.[5]

With Pussy Yoga, you can mobilize your entire body. Not only do you gain fitness, mobility, and a wonderfully sensuous body awareness; you're also be able to move as sexily as you want in your erotic adventures. And that, in turn, makes you more confident, more sensual, and more orgasmic.

If you have any questions or want to get in touch with me and other women who practice Pussy Yoga, join our Facebook group! You can find the link, along with other Pussy Yoga extras, at Coco-Berlin.com/en/pussyyoga.

3. A Happy Pussy

Once you've activated your pelvis and your whole body, we'll take a closer look at the pussy herself. We'll delve into everything that's stopping you from following your sexual instincts freely and without inhibition, surrendering completely in bed, and experiencing life-changing orgasms.

Most women have a hard time feeling or even liking their pussy and recognizing her for what she really is: the most intimate place in their bodies, the part that can experience the most intense sensations, a source of ecstasy— a pleasure center that holds the possibility for deep spiritual connection. Our pussy is also our own personal first aid kit: according to the latest research, it can positively influence and heal both our body and our mind.

With eight thousand nerve endings, the clitoris is an organ whose only function is pleasure and ecstasy. This makes us women unique. (Men, on the other hand, have a "multitool" with only half as many nerve endings, yet they're prouder of it and much more confident about handling it.) Through your newly ignited sensuality, your pelvic floor activation, and your body awareness, your pussy will be able to feel more. You'll be amazed at how your erotic sensitivity increases a thousandfold when all your nerve endings can communicate unhindered with your brain.

4. Life-Changing Orgasms

We're going to look at how our female sexuality works, what we women really need in bed, and why a fulfilling love life is so important to our creativity and power. Then we'll examine the physiology of our orgasms. Once you know what actually happens in your body during sex, you can better navigate your pleasure and ecstasy, reaching previously unknown heights. Sexually, there is much more to experience than most women even imagine.

5. A Sensually Fulfilling Life

Finally, I'll give you some tips on how to cultivate your sensuality in everyday life. With your sensuousness switched on, you'll experience more pleasure and better sex—you will also feel more alive, more vibrant, and more open to the possibilities of life.

It might seem hard to believe—a method for sensuous body awareness and pelvic floor training as life-changing tool? But don't take my word for it. Just try it and experience it for yourself. I always love to see how amazed women are at the rapid and revolutionary effects of my method. The key is right in front of you, hidden inside your own body. The only things stopping you from recognizing it and using it are your old habits and self-image.

I myself started out in life as an anxious, depressed wallflower. I never would have thought it possible that one day, I'd feel good about myself, performing before huge crowds in my own shows, and that later I would help millions of women with my method. I never imagined that I'd spend my life with the man of my dreams, living in the most beautiful places on earth, or that life could feel so effortless and free. Such conceptions simply didn't exist for me. And yet, here I am!

I'm delighted to join you on your journey to a fulfilling love life!

Yours,

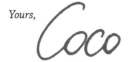

Pussy
Science

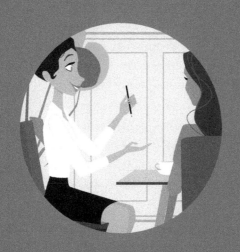

Why Pussy?

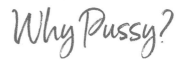

So, why this word? When my German publisher first suggested the title, I was skeptical. My method is about so much more than female genitalia, and apart from that, the word "pussy" is often used in a derogatory sense. On the other hand, what words do we have for our female sex organs that *don't* carry some unsavory connotation or, at best, sound clinical and unsexy?

"Vagina"[6] isn't just a medical term. It stems from the Latin word for "sheath." Our sex organ is therefore defined as being a receptacle for the male sex organ. In her book *The Second Sex*, the philosopher and feminist Simone de Beauvoir argues how, over the course of history, women have been turned into the "second sex" by men. In de Beauvoir's existentialist terminology, this means that man describes himself as the absolute, the essential, the subject, assigning woman the role of "the other," the object. Women are always defined relative to men. The word "vagina" says a lot about our former role in society but is no longer appropriate today.

The body part that brings us the most beautiful sensations and orgasms—that is a place of power, a place of the most intimate connection with ourselves and with our intimate partners, the part to which this book is dedicated—definitely needs a name of its own.

Feminist authors like Eve Ensler, Naomi Wolf, and Regena Thomashauer view the denigration of female sex organs in patriarchal societies like ours as a tool for disempowering women.[7] In my work, and in the culture at large, I still see a great deal of shame about our own sexuality and female sex organs. In ancient cultures, there are more beautiful and fitting names. The Sanskrit word *yoni*, for example, means "source, spring, resting place, container, abode, or nest."

But instead of using a word from a long-gone culture, let alone trying to invent a new one with no existing recognition in our culture, I choose to use the term "pussy" and to make it socially acceptable. The word "pussy" is still used in a derogatory way today, but modern feminists are reclaiming it. Bands like Pussy Riot and Perfect Pussy, the "Pussy Grabs Back" protest movement against the sexism of U.S. President Donald Trump, the *New York Times* bestseller *Pussy* by Regena Thomashauer, and the show *Pussy Terror* by German comedian Carolin Kebekus are all wonderful examples of this trend.

Pussy Yoga stands in this recent feminist tradition. Let's reclaim the word "pussy" and use it with self-confidence. Let's decide for ourselves what the word "pussy" means to us.

"Pussy" has a nice ring to it. Its etymological origin is in the old European term for cat, which has been used to describe girls and women since the seventeenth century.[8] A cat, from a kitten to a lioness, is a great metaphor for this beautiful body part of ours. Cats are soft and cute and know how to command attention. It's inspiring to see how they relax, the way they completely surrender to touch, the confident and smooth way they move— their independence, wildness, and agility. All of that is also the nature of our pussy, whether she is fully activated or still in a state of hibernation.

Through Pussy Yoga, we rediscover our wild, instinctive side. We connect with our animal nature through our bodies, and we become a like a lioness—confident, courageous, sensuous, supple, and strong.

When I use the word "pussy" in this book, I am referring to the entire vulva and the inside of the vagina. While perhaps less anatomically precise, this is generally what our culture commonly understands from the word.

And Why Pussy Yoga?

Yoga is a philosophy and practice that originated in India around 5,000 years ago. Its modern form, as practiced all over the world today, emerged from the mid-19th century. It is characterized by an adoption of Western esoteric ideas, psychology, physical training, and scientific assumptions by English-speaking and Western-trained Indians. This modern yoga represents a new-age approach to life rather than a form of Hindu spirituality. In the feminist movement of the 1990s, women developed their own variations of yoga, focusing on women's wisdom. Today, it is estimated that around eighty percent of Yoga practitioners are women (who were excluded from the traditional form of Yoga in India).[9]

The term "yoga" denotes the integration of body and soul toward becoming one with higher consciousness. In that sense, every path toward self-awareness and consciousness can be described as a "yoga." There are many names for the different yoga paths. The path we are embarking on is the way of the pussy. Pussy Yoga unites body and mind through awareness and movement. It doesn't have a sequence of poses to follow; instead, we experiment with new ways of moving from the pelvic floor. Our focus lies not on perfection, but rather on authenticity, intensity, depth, and vitality. There are no holy scriptures, and there is no master. Your guru is yourself, your body, your pussy. I am sharing a method for you to find your own wisdom and your own power. The treasure you are about to discover already lives within you, and it is something you can only experience for yourself.

Shouldn't Sex Come Naturally?

There seems to be a persistent idea that all of us should be natural masters on the topic of sexuality. Why should that be so? Unlike most animals, we can do more than the bare minimum to procreate. We can become so skilled at sex that it enriches our lives emotionally, spiritually, and intellectually. Just like a master tango dancer, a wise yogi, or a star chef isn't born an expert, a great lover doesn't fall from the sky.

For thousands of years, experts in sexuality from all cultures have been pondering how to refine their artistry to reach higher levels of mastery. Because this knowledge can be shared, we don't all have to start at zero. We can learn from the best instead of fumbling in the dark until we figure out how to surf the big waves. Nobody would dream of taking part in a karate competition without training first, but admitting we want to learn more about sexuality or our pussy is still considered taboo. It's a taboo that we will sweep away with this book. Most women have no idea about the power that lives in their pelvic floor or the power of their orgasms.

I hope you'll enjoy reading this book in the coffee shop or on the subway, and I hope you'll share it on social media and discuss it with your friends. It should be normal for all of us to learn more about our pussies and to talk about them with confidence and curiosity.

Why Are Our Pussies and Pelvic Floors Too Loose and Too Tense?

On the one hand, the circumstances of our lives have changed radically in the last twelve thousand years since we humans settled, and we no longer lead the kinds of lives that our bodies were optimized for by evolution.[10] On the other hand, we have disconnected our bodies from our minds and grown estranged from our instincts and implicit knowledge. As nomadic hunters, gatherers, and fishers, we led active lives. We moved our bodies in ways that trained and utilized them appropriately. Depending on where we lived, we covered great distances. We climbed, dived, hunted, and squatted on the earth to relax or work. We spent our whole lives with our tribes out in nature. Every member of the tribe needed to be capable of doing almost any task, which kept their bodies and minds integrated, fit, and flexible.

Once we started domesticating animals and cultivating plants, we became tied to specific places, and we developed greater specialization. Occupations emerged, and people carried out the same activities over and over again until most of us today, postindustrialization, spend almost all of our time sitting or standing. Compared to our ancestors, we hardly move at all. Thanks to modern forms of transport, we drive instead of walking or running. With the expansion of media, from newspapers, books, and radio to television, the internet, and smartphones, we are not only getting farther and farther away from the present; we're also spending the majority of our leisure time sitting still. We cram our physical movement into a sixty-minute slot at the gym, where we push ourselves to our physical limits.

Today, we spend thirteen hours per day on average sitting. The way we sit on chairs and other furniture seems normal to us, but it's disastrous for our pussy, our pelvic floor, and our abdominal organs. Sitting on chairs as we do only became common within the last two hundred years. Even seated toilets didn't appear in most households until the mid-nineteenth century.[11] The advent of the seated toilet made things even worse for our pelvic floor and abdominal organs. In other words, we no longer lead a *natural* life.

This isn't bad in and of itself because life today is wonderful. I wouldn't want to swap places with my ancestors and give up the opportunity to shape my own life or give up the internet and easy worldwide travel. Besides, we are not helpless; we don't have to live in ways that hurt our bodies. With the insights and practices from Pussy Yoga, you can relearn the skills and abilities that have long since been buried in our civilization. And thanks to the advances of modern civilization, you are getting the latest research and the best tools and tips for a fulfilling love life, all of which our Stone Age sisters could not access.

Another important factor affecting our pelvic floor is that, in contrast to animals and our ancestors, we have become alienated from our body and its inherent instincts. Without this connection, we can no longer handle stress naturally or release it after danger has passed. We are therefore the only animal (with the exception of those we imprison or keep as pets) to have developed ongoing symptoms of stress and trauma. And stress plays a major role in weakening the pelvic floor.[12] There is an unfortunate vicious cycle at play here because people with weakened pelvic floors tend to be more psychologically unstable and prone to stress.[13]

Religious prudishness also played a major role in our alienation from our pelvis. It placed taboos and shame on the natural, beautiful, intimate activity that is sex, as well as on the body parts associated with it. This attitude still paralyzes us today. Although having a lot of good sex is supposedly part of a successful life, today we have less sex than ever in recorded history.[14] Moshé Feldenkrais states that culturally stigmatized areas of the body vanish from our self-image.[15]

And this is exactly where Pussy Yoga comes in. Through conscious practice, you will establish a new neurological self-image, one that moves your pelvic floor back into your awareness.
At the same time, this technique will enable you to free yourself from old, unconscious thought patterns and to experience and express your sexuality according to your own standards.

How I Found the Pelvic Floor and Created This Method

People who are new to my work always ask me, "How did you, as a young woman who had never been pregnant, start thinking about your pelvic floor?" It's only recently that the pelvic floor gained its reputation as "the sex muscle"; before that, it was only known for having something to do with postpartum care and incontinence. People only paid attention to it if something wasn't working.

Although I developed an interest in sex at an early age and was obsessed with becoming a skilled lover, I had never heard about the pelvic floor before I started to research human anatomy as a dancer. I assumed I was using my vaginal muscles for my pussy acrobatics. (By the way, this is a common misconception, and we will clear it up in the chapter called "The Pelvic Floor and the Pussy.")

How the Pelvic Floor Came into My Life

It all started when I decided to learn belly dancing as a teenager in the 1990s. I had a difficult childhood. Emotional and physical abuse led me to dissociate from my body to escape reality. That allowed me to numb my pain and retreat into a fantasy world. I became a shy, depressed child who couldn't see the point in anything. But there were moments when I would be gripped by a mysterious passion and could feel in every fiber of my being that there was hope, and that life could be beautiful. These were moments when a piece of music touched me deeply or when I saw a passionate dancer on TV and sensed that she felt the same as I did. These moments gave me the energy to persist through my depressing reality. One day, on the verge of suicide, I realized that if I had nothing to lose anyway, I was actually free to do anything I wanted. What was the worst thing that could happen? If it all ended in catastrophe or it turned out that I was indeed a total loser, I could always kill myself then. So I decided to leave my wallflower existence behind me. I envisioned a wild and free life full of adventure, romance, and spirit. My inspirations were dancers and femme fatales like Mata Hari, Anita Berber, and Kiki de Montparnasse. I was fascinated by how free they had been and how they had lived life by their own rules—and I wanted to break free from the hopelessness of my small-town life in the same way.

I found a belly dancing video in our city library that I borrowed again and again. I tried out the movements while walking down the street, and later, once my life started to gain more momentum, when I went out to clubs and in my first intimate encounters with boys. Being able to move this way and feel my body gave me confidence. It freed me, step by step, from my old, hated self-image. My new body awareness gave me the eyes to see myself more fully and the strength to stand by this self, to voice my unconventional ideas freely, and to design my life the way I wanted it to be: intellectual, radical, and free.

What Is the Pelvic Floor?

When we humans started walking upright around four to six million years ago, the back wall of our belly became our pelvic floor. The muscles are still the same as they were in our ancestors, but their function has changed. Now the pelvic floor is the lower end of our abdominal cavity, where our digestive and sexual organs are located. It's a combination of muscle and tissue that literally prevents our organs from falling out of our pelvic opening. This pelvic opening is necessarily large so that a baby (with its relatively large head) can pass through at birth.

I kept my belly dancing a secret. I didn't tell anyone why I could move like that—there was something embarrassing about the belly dance cliché. Officially, I was doing ballet, jazz, and yoga; the rest was my natural sexiness. I didn't even set foot in a real belly dance class until 2002, when I moved to Wuppertal to study architecture.

I Became a Belly Dancer

In my first belly dance lesson, I was both fascinated and repelled at the same time. What fascinated me was the mysterious music that touched something deep inside me, like an old memory, a feeling I had known since childhood, vague and impossible to name. It was so intense that I couldn't stop searching for more of it, hoping I would finally figure it out at some point. The feeling contained a hint, a promise, that there was still something hidden in me, still some possibility that I could not yet imagine. But what repelled me, even outraged me, was the amateurism and profaneness of the class. It had nothing to do with my pursuit of beauty and perfection in movement and expression. Everything was "good enough," and you were supposed to just relax and let your belly hang out. As a little control freak, I found that impossible.

During pregnancy, the pelvic floor also carries the baby's weight. Unlike smooth muscles, the muscles of the pelvis are striated, which means we can consciously control, train, and relax them, but only when we learn how to properly locate and activate them.

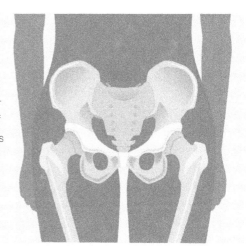

But there was a third element, something I had never found in any other environment before: the solidarity between the women. They all came from different walks of life, but they formed a warm community. They welcomed me with open arms in a way that I'd never been accepted in any group before. It was very touching. I still wore thick emotional armor and hid so much, even from myself, but here I was allowed to just *be*.

In Wuppertal, not only could I badger my Iraqi belly dance teacher, Mona, with all of my questions, I finally had access to better books and CDs too. I devoured everything I could find about the Middle East and dance. I saw my first belly dance shows and found two wonderful mentors in my teachers Isolde Ackermann and Salma Alexandra Abdelhadi. They generously shared their extensive knowledge of Middle Eastern dance with me and supported me on my quest. I researched, danced, and attended all of the workshops I could find, but they only left me hungrier than before. I had this great yearning that nothing I learned could satisfy. I had an inkling that there was still a whole other world waiting for me, but I couldn't grasp it. I wondered why nobody danced the way I imagined in my dreams.

Fast-forward: In the years that followed, I actually became the dancer I had seen in my dreams. I moved to Berlin and developed my own shows, fusing Middle Eastern fantasies with pop culture, tapping into the pulse of the times. I became Germany's most famous belly dancer, dancing on big stages and on national prime-time television. But something was still missing. I didn't know what it was. I had this nagging feeling that I wasn't good enough, that my dancing lacked something essential.

> Pelvic activation makes you feel incredibly feminine and confident enough to show it.
>
> Madeleine, student, belly dance teacher, author

Obsessed with finding that something, I looked for role models from whom I could learn more.

Looking for Clues in Egypt

While researching the countries where belly dance originated, I discovered Egyptian belly dance stars who were as famous as pop stars in the West. They performed with huge orchestras on the stages of five-star hotels and on television, and unlike most Arab women, they lived free, self-determined lives. Sadly, this world of beautiful female expression has all but disappeared since the Egyptian revolution in 2011. With the arrival of a more conservative regime, belly dancing is now banned in those venues.[16]

These women had incredible charisma. They cast a spell on their audiences with moving interpretations of classical Egyptian music and poetry. They gave their viewers goosebumps and brought them to tears of joy, grief, love...and something else I'd never experienced in a performance before: spiritual ecstasy. The feeling they conveyed was more electrifying than any performance or concert I had ever seen before. The Egyptians even have a word for this phenomenon that doesn't exist in any other language: *Tarab*.[17]

I was determined to figure out what these women were doing. Why were they so vibrant, so powerful, so present in their bodies? Sometimes, they would be a sexy femme fatale, then they seemed to enter a trance. Next, they would be playful, joyous, and close. The audience was carried away with them and hung on their every movement.

And the way these women moved! Their movements were smaller but much more intense than those of other belly dancers. They seemed to move straight from their pelvis, straight from their belly, straight from their heart. Sometimes, you wouldn't see any movement at all, but they would build such tension that you could feel it deeply under your own skin.

These women were forces of nature. I sweated; I fevered. I ran hot and cold, feeling new sensations that somehow seemed so familiar to me.

I was filled with passion, and knew I was in the right place to find what I had been looking for all of my life.

At the time, I wasn't exactly spiritual, but in order to understand what those women were doing, only one explanation made sense: these women had a direct connection to something supernatural. They electrified the air and flooded the entire venue with emotion. They were so strong, yet so vulnerable. They revealed so much of themselves without shyness or shame, yet still seemed invincible. I was deeply touched. The spell would not let me go.

I went to their shows, took private lessons, and attended workshops. These Egyptian women are dancers, first and foremost, not teachers. They learn intuitively, without much formal instruction. First, they learn through imitation, the way children learn movement patterns and behaviors from their parents, with the help of mirror neurons.[18] Second, they access subconscious implicit knowledge through their female bodies. Scientists call this "embodied knowledge": it's a biological intelligence, something we've all learned to deny in the West and something we can relearn to use through Pussy Yoga."[19]

I was astonished to discover that this intuitive way of learning worked for me too. I learned their intricate movements from the dancers, but more than that, I learned to open my heart, to feel more deeply, and to trust my feelings. After all, it was my intuition that had led me to them. I started to understand what it meant to be powerful, vibrant, and at home in my own body.

Still, I couldn't figure out how they managed to create those tiny but powerful movements in their hips. These women were doing something different with their pelvis than belly dancers in the West, but I couldn't put my finger on it. I noticed they had a place of power deep inside their pelvis where I felt a void. It was as if I was missing my root, my connection, my essence.

When I was obsessed with femme fatales as a teenager, I experimented with love balls and *Kama Sutra* exercises. I was very familiar with my pussy, so that couldn't be the problem. What was I missing? The Egyptian belly dancers couldn't help me. Did these women not know what they were doing, or were they not willing to share their secrets? It dawned on me that I wouldn't find the answer with their help, nor would I grasp it intuitively on my own. I was completely cut off from something ancient that these women were rooted in.

I had to find it. I knew it would help me answer all my questions and unlock the mystery of life. Who are we? What is that supernatural power, and how can we access it? I knew that it would not only make me a stronger artist and performer; it would also turn me into the powerful, radiant woman I could already sense was inside me.

The feeling that I was on to something fueled me. I wanted to understand my body much more deeply with the help of science, modern body work, and traditional mind-body methods. I wanted to try everything to find the truth about life.

Body Awareness Is the Way

Back in Germany, I began delving into my body, my mind, and my soul with the help of physiotherapy, body work, anatomy, and dance theory. I wanted to understand everything. I noticed that simply understanding my body was already making me a better dancer. Connecting my mind and my body freed my flow of movement. And in turn, everything that made my body strong and supple also freed my mind. At the same time, my dance technique was best when I felt emotionally alive. Our body is the access to our subconscious and the mirror of our soul. The better we understand it, the better we come to know our whole being. The more freely we move, the more liberated we become as human beings. Physical mobility is therefore essential to a fulfilling life.

Connecting with my body in this way was like reuniting with a long-lost and forgotten part of myself. Shedding tears of joy over the reunion and tears for the buried trauma that now dared to come into the light were the order of the day in my work. Every piece of tension or block I dissolved in my body freed something in my mind as well.
I saw more clearly, had more energy, and discovered an increasingly free way of being.
I was on the right path.

In 2006, I started teaching and coaching women. To my great surprise, I found that everything that fascinated me in this work also moved the women who came to me. They not only wanted to learn how to dance; they also yearned to find themselves in their bodies.

Any new discovery I made, I immediately tested on them, and I was thrilled to see that these tools worked for them too. Insights arrived like downloads while I taught. You can look at it spiritually as well as rationally: when we connect with our bodies through our physical sensations, we get access to our "Felt Sense," our implicit body knowledge. In a state of flow, we are also able to combine conscious and unconscious knowledge to create new ideas and insights—and I was usually in a state of flow during teaching! I felt like a dog tracking a scent on a secret trail as I followed my intuition into unknown territory. I forgot who I was and that there was a life outside of the here and now in my studio.

From the outside, teaching was not as glamorous or profitable as my shows, but for me, it was groundbreaking. Watching all of those women transform right before my eyes touched me profoundly. For the first time in my life, I felt the deep satisfaction of having a purpose. I could now create a space where women felt safe and accepted, just as I had felt in my first belly dancing class.

When I completed my degree in architecture in 2007, I had to decide whether to pursue my already successful career as a dancer or to become an architect. Each path would require 100 percent of my focus and energy. It was not an easy decision because, for as long as I could remember, I had been fascinated by both fields. I had pursued architecture with the same passion as dance. I knew that if I became a professional architect, I wouldn't have any more time to research the connections between body, mind, and soul, and I was so close to solving that great mystery. Giving up everything I had worked for seemed the more painful choice, so I decided to go all in on my dancing.

> I am happier and more spontaneous. I feel more freedom in my relationships, and I've lost a lot of inhibitions. My body feels more feminine and attractive, and I can express my intimate emotions better.
>
> Angelica Carmona, psychologist

The Pelvic Floor Is the Key

I threw myself into intensive advanced dance training. At last, here was my chance to spend all day exploring body, mind, and soul, exchanging ideas with other professionals and exploring different areas of contemporary dance and body work. It was my Rolfing therapist who suggested I look more closely at my pelvic floor. I admit, I felt a little attacked. I was a professional belly dancer; we automatically train the pelvic floor—don't we? I had to get to the bottom of this.

I got hold of all the relevant literature on the pelvic floor and started to try out and compare the various approaches. There was a lot of contradictory information, but the methods of Benita Cantieni and Eric Franklin inspired me the most.[20] I trained, researched, and tested everything immediately in my dancing, and bit by bit, I got the feeling that I was finally getting at the key, finally finding my center. I was discovering the thing I was missing in belly dance, its essence, which also seemed to be the key to connecting to my own essence.

The pelvic floor seemed to unlock the answers to all of the questions in my life. Not only did it allow me to develop the same power as the Egyptian dancers; it resolved my fears and doubts and the feeling of not belonging in this world.
The pelvic floor offers direct access to the root chakra, which yogis associate with grounding and a sense of connection. It's something most of us today lack, but we long for it all of the time.

Integrating my pelvic floor gave me an entirely new quality as a woman and a performer in my shows. When I danced, I no longer felt like I had something to prove to those watching me. I just rested within myself and could connect much more deeply with my audience. I was fully present, and could express myself more clearly and authentically. I opened up to a power greater than my small self. It flowed right through me and my audience, electrifying us and permitting me to express things for which there are no words.

My sex life changed too. Not only did I have more desire and strength; I also felt more sensation in my pelvis, as if an entire galaxy of new nerve cells had spung up there. By integrating my pelvic floor and learning to relax my pussy, I discovered for the first time what it felt like to just let go during sex, to just be, instead of performing gymnastics. My students were also enthusiastic! Every woman who finally discovers her own key through my method is deeply touched and astonished that the access to her power has been in her body all along. Pussy Yoga is so important for all of us.

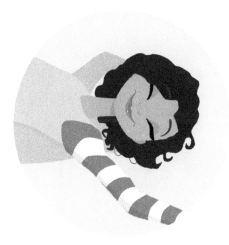

Sensuous Embodiment

Looking back, I've done everything I could in my life just to feel more alive and present—in other words, to fully arrive in my body. It was this sensuous embodiment that enabled me to locate my pelvic floor in the first place. And it's also what has made my method so effective for every woman who has tried it since 2006.

Because my students were so enthusiastic about it, it became the foundation of my work. I've been using it intuitively for a long time, so now I'm excited to see it becoming a trending topic in science. The knowledge I'm presenting to you is therefore based not only on my professional experience but also on that of leading psychologists, therapists, and doctors, as well as the latest scientific discoveries.

What is embodiment? It has to do with "em-BODY-ing." What does it mean to embody yourself? What does it mean to live in your own body? Where are you now? Where is your mind, and where are your feelings? What do you notice in your body now, in this moment? Do you feel you live in your body and know it from the inside out? Or are you more in your head? In front of yourself? Behind? Who are you, anyway? Where does your thinking and feeling arise? What is your mind? Your consciousness? What are our emotions? Your instincts and your intuition? Is there a soul?

Scientists have different answers to these questions compared to philosophers and spiritual teachers. In between, there is a whole range of individual truths. This book exists in the space where the two sides meet, and you can find your way whether you view the world spiritually or in more scientific terms.

Most of us believe our soul is bound to our body while we are alive. When we become human beings, our soul is created in this body or comes into it from somewhere else. We can either believe that it's part of a larger consciousness or that it's made entirely by the body, specifically by our nervous system.

However, the deep connection between body, mind, and soul has long been disputed in Western psychology and medicine. For a long time, medicine looked only at the body, and psychology looked only at the mind. Whereas the ancient philosophers and sages saw interaction and unity, Western scholars created a split. On one side, there was the noble mind with its ideals and morals and, on the other, the sinful body with its needs and drives. The body had to be controlled and mastered by the mind in order for the individual to become a virtuous human being.

> After nine years without contraception, becoming conscious of my feminine energy and the pleasurable relaxation of my pelvis enabled me to conceive our little son.
>
> Dorothee Roldan, Argentine Tango teacher

René Descartes's famous statement, *"cogito ergo sum"* (I think, therefore I am), suggests that the mind is our true self while the body is merely the physical vehicle carrying the mind through life. He placed the mind above the body and feelings, and the majority of people still follow this tradition today.

But we're finally beginning to understand that this intellectual alienation from our bodies—our living, feeling organism and its potential—is one of the main causes of stress and related lifestyle diseases.[21] Our minds clearly aren't the solution to those so-called lifestyle diseases because, even though we intellectually know more and more about ourselves, the World Health Organization documents that these illnesses are on the rise worldwide.[22] Embodiment is therefore essential to a healthy life, both physically and psychologically. That goes double for a fulfilling love life. Without embodiment, there's no sensuality, no full body orgasms; without embodiment, you'll never find your slumbering pelvic floor.

The good news is that all of us can regain access to our bodies. With the right techniques, it's not even difficult—in fact, it's a lot of fun. After the first few Pussy Yoga practices, you'll start to discover the potential for yourself.

How We Develop Body Awareness

How are mind and body connected? And what does that mean for us? Let's take a look at our personal biological creation story from a scientific point of view. From roughly the seventh week of pregnancy, as embryos, we start getting to know our body, and we do this through movement. Our nervous system begins to make contact with our muscle cells. These are stimulated into movement by the nerve cells, which in turn report the status of each muscle to the brain via sensory nerves. This builds the first connections between our motor and sensory nerve pathways.

Initially, we have a vast range of synaptic connections in our brain. The pathways that are activated over and over again by our increasingly well-coordinated movements are the ones that stabilize and settle. This gradually builds our movement patterns. Each individual movement, from waving our limbs to unconscious body processes like breathing, swallowing, and digestion must be practiced. This practice builds a model of our body in the brain, even though we are not yet conscious. At this stage of development, the areas of our brain that will later connect conscious perceptions and reactions are not yet functional.

The primary job of the brain is establishing, maintaining, and changing the relationships between our nerve cells.[23] In other words, our thinking happens in our body. Every thought generates specific arousal patterns in the brain, and through repetition over time, this leads to stabilization of the participating nerve connections, which builds stable pathways. In this way, thinking builds and shapes our brain every day.

As long as we're alive, our brains are capable of making new connections, changing themselves and therefore us. This phenomenon is known as neuroplasticity, and somatic techniques like Pussy Yoga are some of the most effective ways to create these changes. Fundamentally remodeling our self-image in the brain is much easier than trying to change behavior patterns mentally, and it's more effective than perpetual analysis or digging into old, painful memories.[24]

How We Lose Our Body Awareness

After we're born, our primary caregivers' judgments about our thoughts, feelings, and actions play a critical role in the development of our self-image. After all, as babies, we're totally at their mercy. Our lives depend on them remaining well-disposed toward us. For this reason, our self-image contains external components that don't necessarily align with our original body-self. They can reshape or suppress our true potential and may even block our connection with our own body.

As we go through life, more and more discrepancies are added. When our impetuous energy and our urge to move are perceived as disruptive by parents or teachers, they train us to behave according to their rules. We learn that this natural part of ourselves isn't wanted, and we suppress it to avoid punishment or emotional discomfort. We may well become ashamed of our needs and behaviors, and do everything in our power to ensure they never see the light of day.

We gradually learn to suppress the feelings that, as babies, we communicated with our whole body and without shame. We screamed as loud as we could when we were unwell or clapped our hands when we laughed. Without even noticing, we move further and further away from our authentic self, becoming increasingly alienated from ourselves. Our deep need for belonging leads us to cut ourselves off from our physical truth and suppress our needs and feelings.

After the birth of my twins, at last there is movement in my pelvis again. I feel more. I'm much suppler and more flexible, and I have so much more joy and ease in my life.

Michaela Parosanu, teacher

The older we get without recognizing this process, the more we grow away from our origin and the less likely we are to turn back toward our authentic self. After all, the further we've moved, the more afraid we are to lose what we know as our best self. We cling to the life we've built for ourselves, judging others if they choose to live differently. For example, we might perceive confident women who don't stick to society's rules as a threat instead of recognizing them as an inspiration for our own lives.

In my experience, the behavior patterns and characteristics we sacrifice for acceptance are exactly the qualities we secretly long for. This is also one of the reasons why everything we seek already lies within us. Otherwise, the pain of missing it would not be so great.

Envy, therefore, is not a terrible emotion that you should suppress. Instead, it indicates an unmet need, something you're lacking. Whenever you feel envy, it means somebody has or does something that you would like to have or do, someone is living in a way that you are not allowing yourself to live. Suppressing your feelings is about as smart as covering up the dashboard in your car, so you don't have to see the flashing lights. It's better to check the lights and repair your car. All of your feelings are meaningful. They're your inner truth trying to communicate with you. If you push them away, you only cut yourself off from your inner wisdom and intuition, and this takes you further away from yourself.

In Pussy Yoga, as we listen to our body, we will uncover a lot of buried emotions and allow them to reveal themselves in the safe space we create for ourselves. Maybe some have already come up as you read these lines. However scary or uncomfortable they may be, don't worry; you don't need to act on any of them. For now, just acknowledge their existence. We will deal with them later in the book.

Hunting for Treasure in the Subconscious

Based on the way our consciousness develops, all previous experiences and later affective, sensory, and motor impressions are initially stored in the brain without connection to the speech center and cognitive structures. These memories form our subconscious. The body has access to them, but our conscious mind normally does not.

The initial cause for our ongoing adjustment to our environment is the need for survival. As we grow older, we adjust to avoid punishment or social exclusion. We're social beings who are wired to need other humans to survive, so the fear of social exclusion is a real threat. Fear is a particularly strong emotion, and the stronger an emotion is, the stronger the nerve connections associated with it become. That's why connections that help us overcome threatening situations build robust neural highways. When we're children, we therefore develop firmly imprinted survival mechanisms, and we continue to follow these patterns unconsciously into adulthood, even if they only hold us back later in life.

But it's not only fear of punishment that makes such a strong impression on us. We also learn by imitation, through mirror neurons. Mirror neurons are nerve cells in our brains that display the same activity patterns when we watch an activity as when we do it ourselves. So we not only copy the way our parents walk or laugh, but we also unconsciously adopt their values.[25] The patterns we acquire unconsciously shape who we become. This is very effective from an evolutionary perspective, but it might not serve us as individuals today. If you ever find that you're sabotaging yourself in mysterious ways or that you aren't living up to the potential you sense in yourself, you're probably stuck in some old unconscious patterns.

We can access our subconscious with tools like hypnosis, where our conscious mind connects to our subconscious mind and reprograms it. But our conscious mind is also limited and might not know our full potential. There is a better way—a way that is not intrusive and not restricted by our conscious mind. It's the way of the body.

If you want to update your outdated patterns, you'll first need to get to know them and see them with a loving eye. That's a good first step in changing them to favor the person you really are inside.

With Pussy Yoga, you not only train your pelvic floor and upgrade your love life, but you also get powerful tools for rewiring your old patterns, actualizing your self-image, and uncovering your dormant potential. These tools will enable you to create a life that meets your own needs and desires.

Searching for a reason why psychotherapy so rarely succeeds, the psychoanalyst Eugene T. Gendlin studied recordings from thousands of therapy sessions across a variety of methods. He found that neither the therapist nor the method determined therapeutic success; instead, it was something patients did within themselves. The crucial success factor was whether the patient was able to create a connection to something Gendlin called the "Felt Sense." This is our implicit inner wisdom and intuition.

When patients connect with this often unclear but very intense bodily sensation, they can initiate positive changes in themselves by accessing the wisdom of their body. It enables them to assess their lives and problems better, so they can independently overcome crises, traumas, and dysfunctions. Some of us already use our intuition instinctively because this body knowledge is implicit; it's available to all of us. The only thing that cuts us off from it is alienation from our body and a lack of trust in our inner wisdom.[26]

By the way, this does not mean that intellectual analysis is useless. It's incredibly effective, but on its own, it has its limits. In Pussy Yoga, I invite you to open up to your body and a new array of possibilities.

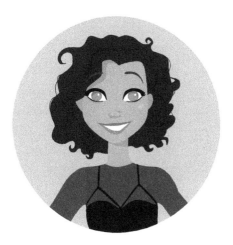

Self-Confidence Is Sexy

Self-confident women are sexy and have better sex, which in turn makes them more confident. But how do you become more self-confident? Spoiler alert: motivational quotes and positive affirmations don't help, but we've found the solution!

As it turns out, thinking you're great doesn't make you happy; it's how closely your self-assessment coincides with reality that matters. In other words, your happiness depends on how well you know yourself.

Our psychological system longs for consistency: it wants freedom from conflict between what we think and feel and what we do and are. It tries to avoid friction caused by inconsistencies because that causes conflict within ourselves.[27] Such conflict leads to stress, depletes our energy levels, and wears us out. Incidentally, we also perceive people with a high consistency as authentic and charismatic.

In a study that compared participants' subconscious sense of self-worth to their conscious perception of self, it became evident that people who see themselves the same way on both conscious and unconscious levels have better psychological health than people who have discrepancies between their conscious and the unconscious self-image. Those who regard themselves well, consciously and subconsciously, also showed the highest happiness levels. Surprisingly, they were closely followed by people who consciously and unconsciously don't think much of themselves. People who appear self-confident on the outside but who are deeply insecure on the inside were about as happy as people who appear hesitant but subconsciously believe they are great, and both groups with this discrepancy were significantly less happy than the former two groups.[28]

This study makes it clear that motivational quotes and affirmations harm insecure people more than they help them because of the inconsistency they create. Knowing and accepting ourselves is the true path to find happiness. And don't worry if you have low self-esteem today. Be honest with yourself, get to know yourself better, and you will improve your self-worth from that healthy place. That's the only way that works.

> If you read an affirmation or a motivational quote that creates an expansive feeling of joy and anticipation in you, then use it. This feeling is invaluable. However, if you read it and feel yourself contracting, then you know you subconsciously don't believe what you've read. Repeating it like a mantra would do more harm than good, increasing doubt in yourself and resistance toward what you're trying to achieve. Either ignore these words completely or use them to take a closer look at your resistance. It can teach you a lot. The practice of Emotional Freedom (in the chapter called "Really Good Sex") will help you unleash the hidden healing potential of unpleasant emotions.

Tip

Your Posture Shapes Your Attitude

How we're feeling shows immediately in our posture. Studies reveal that people who feel satisfied with themselves measurably straighten their spines.[29] It also works in reverse: if we straighten our posture, be it by sustainably integrating the pelvic floor or even by just changing how we carry ourselves temporarily, we feel significantly more courageous. We're more eloquent, assertive, and strong-willed. We also get better results on intelligence tests as well as on tests that assess our willpower, creativity, and perseverance.[30] In addition, scientists have found that others value us more and give us preferential treatment when we stand up straighter.[31]

This interplay between body and mind can be a vicious cycle or a spiral of self-reinforcing positivity. A current study by Dr. Stephen Porges shows that a pelvis in proper alignment not only makes us more self-confident, but also measurably decreases our stress levels.[32] All Pussy Yoga practices will help you to optimally align your pelvis and from there achieve perfect posture.

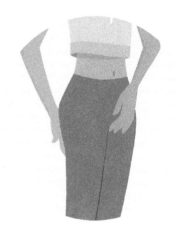

Stress Is Not Sexy

Our nervous system can be divided into the somatic nervous system, which is conscious and controllable, and the autonomous nervous system, which is unconscious and cannot be controlled. The somatic nervous system enables us to consciously perceive our environment through our senses and to perform voluntary action through our muscles. Our autonomous, unconscious, nervous system controls vital functions like heart function, breathing, digestion, and sexual functions. That means our well-being and our sex life depend to a large extent on unconscious processes in our body.

Our autonomous system is divided into two parts that work together as a team: the parasympathetic and the sympathetic nervous systems.

The sympathetic nervous system is activated during stress or strenuous physical activity, enhancing our body's performance. This results in a quicker heart rate, faster breathing, and increasing adrenaline production.
The parasympathetic nervous system, on the other hand, lowers stress levels and helps the body to relax. It ensures we sleep, eat, digest, cuddle, breastfeed, and enjoy sex.

Stress is tension that puts our body into flight, fight, or freeze mode via the activation of the sympathetic nervous system. This not only releases stress hormones and slows our digestion, but it also changes our posture and muscle tone. If this happens often without the corresponding release and relaxation, the tension becomes chronic. In other words, we start to embody our terror. Our body posture, as you know, has a direct effect on our psyche, so over time we enter a vicious cycle. The chronic activation of the sympathetic nervous system can lead to long-term changes in our organs, which in turn can generate psychosomatic illnesses.

Sex and intimacy are very important for our physical and mental well-being because they balance our autonomous nervous system; they are the ultimate stress soothers. That said, in order to have real intimacy and good sex, we women absolutely require the right mood and a feeling of safety. Our autonomous nervous system needs a certain balance to allow arousal.[33]

Only when we feel safe in intimacy can our body release oxytocin, the love hormone, which enables orgasms. If our body feels stressed, it prevents this release.[34] All of this happens unconsciously; you can't simply flip a switch inside your autonomous nervous system. However, you can indirectly influence your nervous system with conscious relaxation, as you will learn through Pussy Yoga.

Simple Doesn't Mean Easy

The biggest killer of a satisfying love life isn't lack of technique. According to science, it's stress. Usually, we rush through our lives, moving from one task to the next, barely even noticing we're stressed.

This is something I have to keep reminding myself of as well because, like most of us, I was raised with the attitude that life is full of obligations to be met. Having checked one thing off the list, the next one is already waiting until one day everything is perfect, and we're allowed to rest at last. Resting before we reach this perfection is laziness, and it doesn't work anyway because our guilty conscience plagues us, preventing us from truly letting go.

What's worse, whenever we dare to relax for a minute, we're hit with motivational quotes about leaving our comfort zone to keep growing because, as we all know, standing still is regressing. In reality, this is the wrong kind of motivation. It puts the cart before the horse, and as I'm sure you know from your own experience, it's doomed to fail. Then we stress out even more as we beat ourselves up for our lack of discipline.

After all, stress is not only caused by actual threats like impossible dead-lines but also by negative thoughts that we turn on ourselves. Stress has been proven to weaken our pelvic floor.[35] It disrupts our hormonal balance and causes sleep disturbances, which in turn increases stress levels. It's a vicious cycle. How can we break free? Timeouts are all very well and good, but the effect doesn't last long. Before long, we're caught in a negative feedback cycle again.

> With Pussy Yoga, we can escape this hamster wheel by learning to consciously relax and then act from a state of ease. Studies show that our true power comes from a rested state. When we're relaxed and centered within ourselves, we can access passion, inspiration, and the motivation and energy to pursue our goals.[36]

That said, even Pussy Yoga can create stress if you pressure yourself to obtain perfect pelvic floor mastery and mind-blowing orgasms within a specific time frame. Simply put, if you forget our motto that "the journey is the destination," and turn your pleasure sessions into tasks that you have to do—so that, at some point in the future, when you've really earned it, you'll be allowed to have some real fun—you're going into the wrong direction. As the piano pedagogue Rudolf Kratzert states, "Strained practice produces poor skill."[37] That is true in all disciplines, but it especially applies to Pussy Yoga.

So please take the focus off performing and instead concentrate on sensing and experiencing. Sensing is more important than doing. If you consistently practice sensing inside yourself, you'll have better results from the book, and you'll learn an invaluable skill for life: you'll be able to control your mind and relax in every situation life throws at you.

As with so many things in life, Pussy Yoga isn't about knowing what is right intellectually. As Derek Sivers puts it, "If information was the answer, then we'd all be billionaires with perfect abs."[38] The key lies in our ability to use information and act accordingly. In our case, that means consciously cultivating a relaxed, sensuous attitude in our lives.

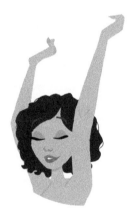

Making the Connection between Body and Mind

Before you can activate and use specific muscles in your pelvic floor, you need to become aware of them. Most of us are so alienated from our pelvic floors that, in the beginning, it takes a lot of mental energy to strengthen the conscious connection between our pelvic floor and our nervous system. Each time you practice, your body awareness will become finer and more differentiated. We'll use the principles of ideokinesis, meaning we start by imagining the movements we want to make or the muscles we want to activate.

> By focusing on releasing all tension in the pelvis and from there imagining doing the practices in your mind first, your nervous system will gradually create connections between those muscles and your conscious mind. This will enable you to use previously unknown muscles to do exactly what you want.

In my experience, this is the only way to really understand your pelvic floor, gain full sensuous awareness of it, and deliberately control it. This is often the missing element in conventional pelvic floor training, which makes it so boring and fruitless.

If you're too focused on actively doing something and desperately tighten whichever muscles you can find, it's possible that you'll train your pelvic floor in the wrong way or even activate completely different muscles. Then it becomes impossible to truly experience the pelvic floor network from the ground up and, from there, to work it effectively.

It's as Moshé Feldenkrais says, "Only when you know what you're doing can you do what you want."[39]

In our approach, less is more. Overzealous or improper training can lead to problems, and relaxation is a valuable skill to master in today's stressful world. After working with thousands of women, I know that this refined, delicate approach is not easy, especially if you already have problems with your pelvic floor and want a quick solution. That's when it's crucial not rush ahead and tighten the wrong muscles. Instead, take your time to carefully get to know this part of your beautiful body, with all its intricacies. This is how you turn your pelvic floor into the powerful centerpiece of your body that it can be, and that it must be for a fulfilling life. The great thing about our approach is that you'll start to enjoy the benefits before you even begin to perceive or move the muscles and bones of your pelvis.

Taking Time for Yourself

From my observations, I know that we women aren't particularly good at taking time for ourselves. If you aren't following an instructor, a video, or an audio program, you'll probably rush through the practices in this book so you can feel like you've made progress. Maybe you even stop early to deal with laundry or emails. You could also be one of those women who will read the book but won't do the practices at all, leaving them until later—and later never comes. If this sounds like you, I have a tip to preempt this self-sabotage. Set aside some time, say thirty minutes, and use a timer (like the one on your phone) so you can dedicate yourself fully to the pleasure of these practices during your precious me time.

After only thirty minutes of engaging with the practices in this book, you'll have a new body awareness, better alignment, and a refined perception of your pelvis. Even if we can't feel anything moving, our muscles respond when we imagine movement.[40] The practices not only train your pelvic floor; they also increase your mental strength and your ability to focus in your daily life. Soon you'll notice how, day by day, you gain more control over the muscles in your pelvic floor and how they start to automatically activate and strengthen in your everyday life. Trust is an important prerequisite for Pussy Yoga. Imagine the movements in your body from the inside and feel how, little by little, something in your pelvis awakens and moves.

The mental aspect of our Pussy Yoga training has even more benefits. It trains the connection between the left and right sides of the brain, helping us to connect intellect and creativity in our lives. When we become aware of the processes in our bodies, we promote neural connections between the most primitive parts of our brain (brainstem and

Simply looking at a clock isn't as effective, because then you won't be able to keep your full attention on the practices. Select a pleasant alarm tone that is gentle and doesn't make you jump in fright. We're at a spa, after all, not at a gym. If you prefer to practice without a timer, and this works well for you, that's perfect. The timer is for women who find it difficult to take time for themselves.

I've recorded some practices for you at Coco-Berlin.com/en/pussy-yoga. There, you'll also find bonus materials to help you integrate Pussy Yoga into your daily life. If you want video guidance, join me on SensuousWorkout.com or in the premium membership area of EssenceBellydance.com limbic system), which are responsible for unconscious bodily processes, instincts, and emotions, and the more recently developed part (neocortex), which is responsible for conscious action and thinking. This integration makes us more present, and the practices have an effect on us that is similar to a deep meditation.[41]

The best part about our conscious approach is that you can get rid of all of the bad movement habits you may have acquired throughout your life. For example, when you were told to contract your pelvic floor during yoga or Pilates without really knowing where it was, you may have learned to contract the wrong muscles. The only thing you need to do is set aside everything you learned before and start with a clean slate to build a new, relaxed, and natural connection with yourself and the wisdom of your wonderful body.

A Step-by-Step Guide to Complete Integration of the Pelvic Floor

In the practices that follow, we'll focus on specific images and directions of movement to enable the pelvic floor and the rest of our musculoskeletal system to integrate and connect, creating an effective, healthy network. With this ideokinetic approach, we allow our bodies to find the optimal natural movement without our old habits getting in the way. It enables us to move freely and without effort. This is also what makes us capable of any action. Only when complex movements like walking and swimming can occur automatically (without us having to activate each muscle individually) do we have enough capacity in the brain to think about where we are going and why.

The same applies to the pelvic floor. Once the necessary muscles are integrated and work together automatically, we can move our bodies the way we like to get all the satisfaction we want in bed. Then we don't have to think about technique and can surrender to the passion of the moment.

In order to empower as many women as possible to find intuitive access to their pelvic floor, I've developed a system of various practices and entry points for finding and activating the pelvic floor. I encourage you to try them all playfully, with curiosity and lightness, because as soon as you fixate, you stifle the process. This is why the individual practices are often split into several parts.

★ Start with Part 1 and do the practice until you're satisfied. If you feel like you aren't progressing, let the exercise rest until your next session and move on to the following practice.

★ If you're satisfied and feel like you're on the right track, then move on to Part 2 of that same exercise to deepen it. Go on until you've mastered the entire practice. Later, you'll trust your body and intuitively select the right practices and intensities.

Pussy Yoga helps you to build a close relationship with your body and pelvic floor. Once you have this connection, you always know what your body needs in order to be at its best.

How to Practice

The practices you'll find here are not designed to be a strenuous workout. They should be as relaxing as a spa break. This is your time to spend with yourself. It benefits your body, your mind, and your soul. You'll know you're doing it right when, after each session, you feel rejuvenated and look like you've just come back from vacation. Depending on your schedule, your sessions could last anywhere from five to sixty minutes daily. The more time you invest, the better the effects.

Because we're working holistically, it's impossible to train too much. Nevertheless, if your muscles should ever feel strained, take a few days' rest. If you're training consistently, a break of a few days could also help you progress because it gives your body the opportunity to integrate the new patterns it has learned.

I recommend you take time to connect with your body and pelvic floor every day. You might try right after you wake up and just before you go to sleep.

Start with fifteen minutes in the morning and five minutes at night. You'll soon notice how good it is for you, and maybe you'll extend the time. Or how about five minutes every morning and thirty minutes a few times a week? Whatever you pick, stick with it and don't let it slide. Your future self will thank you.

Even when you don't really have time, squeeze in a few minutes here and there. The training has a slow but lasting positive effect on your psyche and your mind. You'll become more balanced and gain a new perspective on yourself and on life. With your new outlook on life, you'll probably be able to set better priorities, so new windows of time will open up for you. I've noticed that the quality of my life goes down when I skip my conscious time with myself and my body. Slowly but surely, I become unbalanced, inattentive, and unclear. This affects everything from my work to my relationships. The trick is to stay consistent with the practices and in contact with yourself in good times and in bad.

Most of us start new habits when we feel the need to change something in our lives. The starting point is dissatisfaction, but as soon as our situation improves, other things seem more attractive and important. Then we become careless, dropping our new habits before they can really establish themselves. We think we've got it all sorted out now, so we don't need them anymore, but little by little, the effects fade away without us noticing. Once we feel really bad again, we start from scratch. This means we never get past the limit we set for ourselves because every time we start to feel a bit better, we let everything slide.

So please keep your Pussy Yoga practice active. Keep exploring and expanding after you already feel amazing. Don't stay at the surface level; there is so much more!

The Best Place to Practice

Look for a beautiful and private place where you can let go. Choose clothing that feels good and allows you to move. You can practice on a carpet, a yoga mat, a blanket, or a combination of these. Personally, I love a shag rug or a yoga mat layered with a really soft blanket. I spread them out completely to make a large, soft nest. This allows my body and my senses to let go and indulge. It's your personal wellness time, so make it beautiful for yourself. Treat yourself as you would want to be treated in a luxurious spa. Enjoy calmly and pleasurably connecting with your body, your mind, and your soul.

> Play with doing all of the practices in bed in the morning or evening as well. They're also a perfect remedy if you can't sleep at night.

Once you're familiar with the practices and know your favorites, you can use them as you like. Create your own sequence or fit them into your daily routine. With some modifications, almost all of the practices can be done while sitting, squatting, standing, lying down, or walking—in other words, anywhere and anytime. If there are people around, you can close your eyes or just stare into the distance. No one will notice what you're doing.

I've done these practices on public transport, in airplanes, and in the car. It's like a minivacation or a meditation retreat, after which you arrive at your destination completely refreshed and aligned. Reading a book, chatting online, or answering emails doesn't have the same effect. Other good places to practice are restaurants, movie theaters, boring meetings, or waiting in line, especially if you're in a hurry, and it doesn't seem to be moving forward.

Many of the practices give you an amazing sense of authority, clarity, and presence, especially when you consciously relax the pelvic floor. You may want to use them for public speaking or important meetings and negotiations.

You can do all of the practices on your own anywhere. You don't need any tools or accessories. They will become your personal toolkit that you'll always have with you. You can use them to relax, center yourself, fill up with fresh energy, ignite your sexual power, or just have a good time.

Make Pussy Yoga a highlight of your day. Just like sex, you shouldn't turn it into a duty. Allow yourself to enjoy it.

Why Feeling into Your Body and Observing the Effects Is So Important

Make sure you take the time to notice what you feel in your body when I mention it in the practices, or whenever you need to. Sensing your body isn't simply a relaxation exercise you can ignore. Yes, it's relaxing and feels good, but more importantly, it's the moment when your nervous system integrates the information from the practices, so it's an essential part of practicing. Noticing the effects trains your brain and sharpens your senses. It heightens your interoception, which is the assessment of inner processes in your body, bringing you closer to your intuition and your Felt Sense. It also increases your sense of balance and your proprioception, which is the perception in your muscles, your joints, and your body position.[42]

This will help with self-actualization and ultimately increased self-confidence. Feeling into your body is an essential part of the Pussy Yoga way.

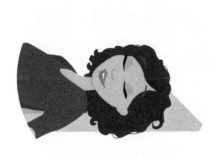

Sensuous Pussy Yoga Training

Waking Up the Pelvic Floor

These first practices will help you to become aware of your pelvic floor. Like explorers, we'll discover new territory and draw an internal map. This is how, bit by bit, we become fully conscious of our body and our pelvic floor. Once you become fully aware of your pelvic floor, you can consciously use it, train it, and enjoy it.

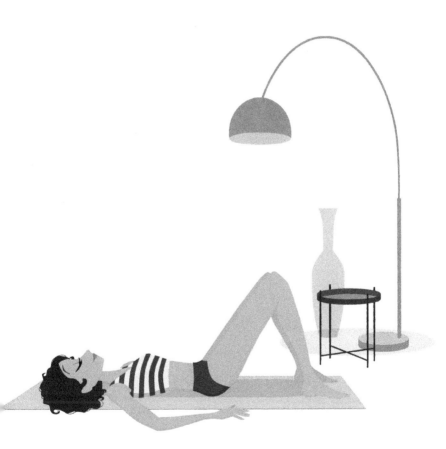

PRACTICE 1: Feeling the Pelvic Bones

We'll start with the pelvic bones, which hold the edges of the pelvic floor. In Pussy Yoga, we want to achieve dynamic movement with these bones. This is the most effective way to activate our pelvic floor and then connect it with the surrounding muscles so it comes into its full power as their centerpiece. Let's begin by locating the pelvic bones in our body. Our pelvis is formed by our two hip bones and our sacrum. The sacrum is part of the spine; more specifically, it's the place where the spine crosses the pelvic ring. Under the sacrum, at the end of our spine, hangs our little tailbone (coccyx). This little piece is often underestimated, but it plays an important role in the biomechanics of our body structure because it's connected with the entire pelvic floor.

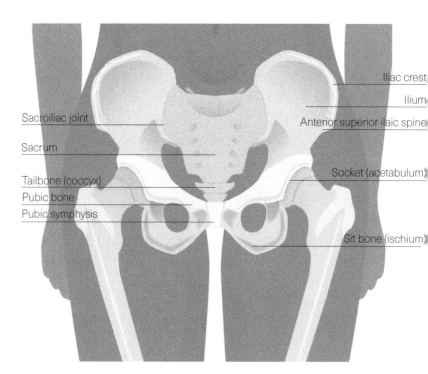

Iliac crest
Ilium
Sacroiliac joint
Anterior superior iliac spine
Sacrum
Socket (acetabulum)
Tailbone (coccyx)
Pubic bone
Pubic symphysis
Sit bone (ischium)

1 We start in our basic lying position. Lay down on your back, bend your knees, and place your feet in front of the pelvis, maintaining a long, relaxed spine. Then find your pelvic bones with both of your hands. We'll start with the anterior superior iliac spine, which are the two bones found to the right and left of your lower belly. These are what we refer to as our "hip bones," and they may stick out a little if you're lying down.

Once you've found them, you can grab them quite firmly to see how far into your body you can feel them. Don't worry—you can't hurt yourself by exploring the area around them; a good massage therapist does the same thing. Next, follow these bones to the sides of your body and feel them all the way to the spine. You'll need to lift your pelvis to do so.

2 As the pelvic bones approach the spine, they form the sacroiliac joint with the sacrum. Yes, this is in fact a joint, and it means your pelvis isn't as stiff as most of us imagine. We will bring a lot of movement into it soon. Feel your way around this area, and try to grasp the long seam of the sacroiliac joint in its entirety. Then take your arms out to your sides, and let your pelvis float back down to the floor.

3 Place your hands on your iliac crests at the front once more, and follow them down in the other direction toward your pubic bone. How far can you feel your bones before they're covered by the strong tendons, muscles, and tissue of your groin? Follow the line of your groin until you find your pubic bones. Their Latin name is *os pubis*. The pubic bones form a joint as well where both hip bones meet in a symphysis, which is a fibrocartilaginous fusion between two bones. Take time to feel the pubic bones and the joint from all sides. Again, you can go pretty deep here.

4 Now follow the pubic bone further down to your sit bones (ishia), which are the two bones you might feel if you sit on a hard chair. Circle them with your fingers so you understand their position in your body.

5 Then take your arms out to your sides and touch the sit bones from the sides. Continue to follow the bones until you're back at the spine and sacroiliac joint.

6 From the sacroiliac joint, follow the spine all the way down until you come to its very end. This last section of your spine is the coccyx or tailbone, the remnant of our former tails.

7 Finally, place your hands back by your sides, and take some time to observe the sensations in your pelvis and your body. How do you perceive your pelvic skeleton in your body now? How does your pelvis feel? How is your mood?

Tip

You can do this practice any time during the day without even touching your body.

1. Where do you feel your pelvic bones? Track them mentally and imagine your pelvis as a whole as well.

2. Visualize doing this practice while shining a golden light on your pelvic bones.

3. Feeling your pelvis as a whole makes you more present in your body, and that can be irresistible. Try it sometime with your partner or when you're flirting.

Your pelvic floor essentially consists of three layers. Let's explore these together.

Outer Layer

The outer or first layer is located between the pubic bone and the tail-bone. It circles around the openings of the urethra, vagina, and anus like an infinity symbol. The muscles cross each other at the perineum. This layer is the one most women know well. You use this layer every day to hold in urine and feces. Usually it's well trained, and in some women, it may even be quite tense. Because they're not aware of the rest of their pelvic floors, most women confuse this first layer with the entire pelvic floor. This is what they clench when they try to activate their pelvic floor in yoga, Pilates, or during conventional pelvic floor training.

This can be dangerous because it gives them the illusion of training their pelvic floor by closing only the sphincter muscles. They miss their chance to find their entire pelvic floor network, the true center of their musculoskeletal system. In addition, training the first layer excessively can bring the tailbone too close to the pubic bone, narrowing the bottom of the pelvis. This causes the first layer of the pelvic floor to tense up while the pelvic floor muscles that really matter hang slack above them.[43] Most of us don't need to train the first layer. Instead, we need to focus on conscious perception and relaxation. To be absolutely sure you understand, let's spend some time getting to know the first layer properly.

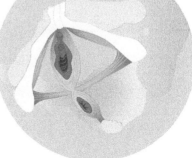

PRACTICE 2: Locate the First Layer of the Pelvic Floor

1 Place one finger on your tailbone at the end of the spine and one on your pubic bone. Between them is the first layer of your pelvic floor. Now place one finger on your perineum, the place between the vagina and the anus; this is where the fibers cross to form the infinity symbol.

2 Imagine you have eyes that open and close at the entrance to your urethra, your vagina, and your anus. Play with winking with each eye and see how finely you can coordinate these contractions. Wink gently and firmly. Observe whether you can feel the muscle as a whole too. Take your time with this practice, and then relax deliberately. It helps to imagine that the muscle you've worked sinks down toward the earth, deeper and deeper with every out breath.

3 Now close each eye very tightly, one after the other, from front to back, and feel how the muscles contract more and more. Hold this tension as long as it feels good, but don't forget to keep breathing. Maybe you can feel how your pubic and tail bones come together. Then release the whole muscle slowly and completely. Observe how long it takes until it's totally relaxed.

4 Next, try the practice in the other direction. Afterward, relax again.

As soon as you're sure you know this layer well and can activate it when you wish, you won't need to do this practice again. In Pussy Yoga, we'll focus on the vital third layer.

It's important to make sure you let go of this first layer when doing any of the following practices in this book. As long as this layer is activated, you'll have a hard time finding the other layers. Use Practice 3 to relax between exercises and anytime you want to relax throughout your day.

PRACTICE 3: Completely Relax the First Layer

Maybe you notice that it isn't easy for you to release the tension in the first layer completely after these practices. You may also notice during your day that you unconsciously tense the first layer when you're stressed or don't feel well. Don't worry; it isn't bad thing. It's your body's way of telling you something is off. If you notice it happening, embrace it, because now you have the opportunity to act on it and decrease your stress level with the following practice.

1 Consciously decide to let go of the first layer. Imagine it sinking toward the earth. Breathe in, and feel this layer; breathe out, and let go even more.

2 If you're not feeling relaxed yet, keep going. Imagine your first layer inflating like an inner tube when you breathe in and deflating when you breathe out. Do this practice for a few minutes. Then take it with you into your everyday life.

Middle Layer

This sheet of muscle and tissue stretches like a taut cloth at the front in the triangle between the two sit bones and the pubic bone. In almost all of the practices in this book, it will activate appropriately by itself.

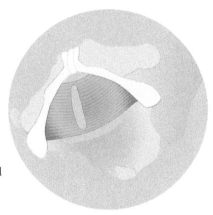

PRACTICE 4: Locate the Middle Layer of the Pelvic Floor

1 Reach in between your legs all the way down to your sit bones and massage them a little. Now move your fingers along these bones to the front of your body until you reach your pubic bones. They're joined together by cartilage. Between the sit bones and the pubic bone joint is the second layer of the pelvic floor. The middle of this layer contains a slit for your vagina and urethra.

2 Imagine that this layer is stretched like a firm cloth between your bones; engage the muscle by imagining you're pulling the cloth together toward its center. It may take some time before you feel anything. Imagine this continuous pull and stay with it while you keep breathing calmly. Once you notice some tension building in the front of your pelvic floor, like moving the pubic bones together, you're on track to find the second layer of your pelvic floor.

3 If you're a little more advanced, this layer will feel more like a plate, and you'll eventually notice a connection to your abdominal wall, somewhere between your pubic bone and your navel. In some women, you can see a horizontal line there; this is the linea

arcuata. In the Essence of Bellydance and the Sensuous Dance Workout, we use this spot to make the backward movements of our hips even more juicy. Later, when you engage your middle layer like that, you may find that your entire abdominal wall tightens, your pelvis aligns, and your lower spine stretches.

> You can do this practice from time to time, but please remember to consciously relax this layer as well.

PRACTICE 5: Relax the Middle Layer

1 Feel your second pelvic floor layer in your body, and consciously let it go. Imagine it filling with fresh air as you breathe in, and let it drop down as you breathe out.

2 Now imagine using a garden hose to let soft, warm water run through this layer. Feel the water moisten, soften, rinse, and refresh your second layer. Allow yourself to release all tension and let go.

3 Feel how the rest of your body relaxes deeply as well. If you like, you can use the imaginary garden hose for your entire body now. Completely rinse and refresh yourself.

Inner Layer

The third layer is the most important muscle group in our pelvic floor. The levator ani is like a fan-shaped funnel with many different parts. This muscle network stretches between your tailbone, your pubic bones, and the two sit bones. Its exact structure is still disputed among specialists, but you don't need to worry about these details. [44] For healthy and effective pelvic floor training, we'll concentrate on feeling into and activating the levator ani as an entire muscle network. My work has proven the effectiveness of this approach.

Most of the practices in this book are dedicated to this innermost layer. We'll approach it slowly in the following practices, but first, we'll clear up some common misunderstandings about the pelvic floor.

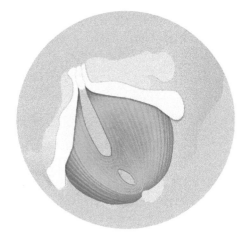

The Pelvic Floor and the Pussy

Your pussy herself is not a striated muscle that you can consciously activate. In exercises that direct you to squeeze your pussy, you're not training your pussy directly. Instead you're working on the pelvic floor muscles immediately surrounding your vagina, especially the first layer and the musculus pubococcygeus (commonly known as the PC muscle). The PC muscle is only a small part of the levator ani, the third layer of the pelvic floor. Therefore, exercises in which you activate your pussy only train a fraction of the pelvic floor complex.

Calling these exercises (and any exercises with weights) "pelvic floor training" is misleading. On the one hand, this can mean that women who believe they're doing something good for themselves instead let their pelvic floor slacken. On the other, strenuous training with weights has been shown to lead to vaginal cramps, bladder problems, and pain during sex.[45]

Biomechanics and movement expert Katy Bowman has also found that any pelvic floor training that shortens the pelvic floor muscles (which is always the case when we focus on the vagina) brings the pelvic bones into a rigid and unnaturally tight position. Eventually, this causes the pelvic floor to sag, so it can't stretch and activate in the best way for the body. Any pelvic floor training that only works with contraction and doesn't include dynamic movement and pelvic floor stretching can be counterproductive or even harmful.

In Pussy Yoga, we train the pelvic floor holistically and dynamically. This is a powerful way to make your pussy fit, firm, strong, and sensitive. In addition, all of your female organs and your bladder get a natural lift. All of these practices help your pussy to function naturally during sex, ensure good circulation, and create better neural connections to the brain, which is crucial for good sex and satisfying orgasms. And they do much more than that.

In Pussy Yoga, we actively integrate our pelvic floor into our natural movement, which is how evolution optimized it. That's a better approach, not only for our love life, but for everything else as well: our entire body aligns from the inside out, and our movements become more effective and efficient. You'll notice this right away in any physical activity: you'll have more fun running, working out, shopping for hours, strolling around museums, taking flights of stairs with ease, and sitting upright without strain.

To make sure you use the Pussy Yoga exercises to train your entire pelvic floor, please pay attention during your practice. You shouldn't feel like your pussy is tensing in any way. To be able to activate the masterpiece that is your pelvic floor, your pussy must be able to relax. You can experiment with weights or jade eggs[46], but in order to connect to all of the intricate layers of your pelvic floor, I recommend that you master all of the practices in this book first.

Anatomy of the Vagina

The vagina stretches from your inner labia up to your uterus. In an adult woman, this stretchy tube is about three to five inches long and consists of muscle and connective tissue.[47] The vagina lies approximately in the pelvic axis and crosses the pelvic floor here.[48] When it's not being stretched, it's flattened by the paracolpium, a dense part of the inner pelvic fascia that flattens the vagina between the bladder and rectum. The anterior and posterior walls touch and enclose the lumen (the inside space) of the vagina. They form an H-shaped gap, allowing for great unfolding without great tension. In addition, there are transverse folds in the front and back of the vaginal wall, which increase sensation during sex and at the same time allow stretching for the baby moving through during labor.[49]

Once you've experienced your pelvic floor as a whole, we'll move on to specific pussy exercises. But for now, let's just locate it from within and learn to relax it.

PRACTICE 6: Drop the Pussy—Deep Relaxation

1 Lie down and let your breath flow. Consciously relax. Listen to your pelvis and try to feel your pussy from within.

2 Breathe in; feel your pussy. Breathe out; let it sink toward the earth, deeper and deeper. Once you're relaxed, let go even more. Soften even more.

If you're used to holding a lot of tension in your pelvis, you may feel a little bit dizzy, but keep going and surrender to this new experience. You have nothing to lose except your inhibitions and control issues.

If you find yourself stressed out in everyday life, use this practice and explore what's going on in your emotional world. Let go and let yourself be wild. During sex, if you feel like you want to force your orgasm, let go and keep letting go. Let the orgasm come to you. Once you're used to this feeling, do the exercise any time you want. You'll notice that you relax more and feel more, becoming more open, confident, and sexy.

Tip

What About the Butt Muscles?

Your butt muscles have three layers, and many women automatically tense them when trying to find their pelvic floor. In order to make sure you find and work your pelvic floor, consciously keep your glutes soft in all of our practices (unless the practice requires that we consciously activate them).

To anchor your butt muscles in your consciousness, go ahead and tense them as tightly as you can for as long as you can. Now let them go slowly and try to let go of all built-up tension.

Your butt muscles are important counterparts to your pelvic floor. They work together to hold your pelvic bones and the sacrum in the right position. The butt muscles are therefore essential in keeping your pelvic floor flexible and fit. Later on, we'll train them consciously with squats (see Practice 51).

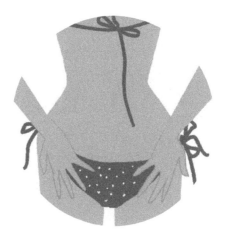

What About the Abdominal Muscles?

It's important that you keep your abs relaxed during each exercise. Our bellies are often very tense because we unconsciously suck them in all the time. This squeezes our organs, so they no longer work as well as they could. It also strains the diaphragm, limiting our ability to take a full breath, so our pelvic floor becomes slack or chronically tense. Sadly, the belly always comes first in surveys when women rank the parts of their body they dislike.[50] Relaxing your belly can therefore be a wonderful exercise in self-love. Once your pelvis aligns through pelvic floor training, your belly will automatically become slender in a healthy way.

PRACTICE 7: Belly Massage

Stroke your belly with your hands. Feel the skin over it. Then observe from the inside how your belly perceives your touch. See if you hold tension and explore how you feel about that. Massage your belly. Send an inner smile to it and the organs inside that keep you alive.

Do this exercise whenever you lie down and relax somewhere. You might be on your sofa or outside sunbathing. Do it calmly and lovingly. If you feel like it, explore what's going on in your emotional world.

Tip

PRACTICE 8: Deep Relaxation for Pelvis and Organs

If you notice that you're tense and that the stress of the day is still in your body, do this exercise before you begin your Pussy Yoga practice.

1 From the basic lying position, feel your body on the ground, your feet, your hips. Follow your spine to the ribs, the shoulder blades, the head, and then the arms.

2 Let everything feel heavy and drop toward the earth. Take one deep breath for every body part. Now consciously let your pelvic bones sink deep into the earth. Let go more with every breath.

3 Then let everything you know in your pelvis and belly drop into the earth: pussy, womb, ovaries, small intestine, large intestine, bladder. Continue on to the kidneys, adrenal glands, stomach, lungs, heart. Keep going again and again through all of your organs until you've released all tension. If you like, you can talk to your organs, saying something like "Thank you for all you do to keep me alive. You can rest now."

Tip

We hold so much tension in our organs that relaxing like this can bring up suppressed emotions. Allow it all and know you don't have to solve anything right now. Everything that comes up is okay and allowed. This practice is also a great tool for falling asleep.

Pelvic Floor and Breath

In order to master your pelvic floor, it's important that you understand the connection between the pelvic floor and breathing.

In the beginning, the following practices require a lot of sensitivity and imagination, so don't worry if you can't imagine or feel everything right away. Trust the process and keep going. Soon, it all will become natural and easy for you. You're learning a powerful tool to relax and recharge, anytime and anywhere.

The pelvic floor is a muscle network that stretches throughout your pelvis between your pubic bones, your tailbone, and your sit bones. You can imagine it like a bowl made from a firm but slightly stretchy material. This bowl forms the lower part of your abdominopelvic cavity, which contains all of your reproductive and digestive organs. The upper side of this cavity is the diaphragm, which opens like a parachute. The cavity is circled by your front and transverse abdominal muscles and your back muscles, so it's very flexible.[51] Above the diaphragm sit your lungs and your heart.

The lungs don't breathe by themselves because they're not made of muscle. All of the work is done by the diaphragm with help from the intercostal muscles between your ribs. This is how it all works together: when you breathe in, your diaphragm pulls down, your chest expands, and your lungs widen, so air naturally flows in. The pull of the diaphragm pushes the organs in the abdominal cavity down, so they seek more space and expand your elastic abdominal wall to find it. At the same time, they push against the pelvic floor, stretching it downward a little. When you breathe out, the diaphragm stretches upward and pushes the air out of the lungs, which allows your organs to come back up. This flattens your belly and allows the pelvic floor to relax back into its original place.

PRACTICE 9: Integrated Pelvic Floor Breathing

Take at least five minutes to go through the following sequence.

1 Visualize the anatomy of your body as just described. Observe how breath flows into you and out of you. The breath comes and goes by itself; you don't have to do anything. Let it flow. The way it is right now is just right.

2 Now imagine your diaphragm inside of you, and try to sense it in your body. To better understand this internal movement, you can use your hands to help: move them down in front of your rib cage when you inhale, and move them up when you exhale.

3 Then focus on the rise and fall of your belly in connection with the movement of your diaphragm. Try observing both the diaphragm and belly as they work together.

4 Next, place your attention on the pelvic floor area between your sit bones, your pubic bone, and your tailbone. See what you can observe there. If you need a reminder, you can feel for these bones in your body so your nervous system knows what it's supposed to pay attention to. Then your body also gets the signal to loosen and realign there.

5 Now try to feel your lungs and your entire abdominopelvic cavity all at once.

I know this anatomical conception of the diaphragm and abdominopelvic cavity is difficult for most people, but once you master it, you'll have a better foundation for connecting to your pelvic floor. You'll also have a wonderful tool that enables you to use your full respiratory potential to oxygenate your body completely, massage all organs, get full blood circulation, and keep your lymphatic detoxification fit. Plus, you'll learn how to breathe deeply in order to relax and soothe your autonomous nervous system in stressful situations. Deep, conscious breathing will also give you more sensuality and deeper orgasms.

Pussy Yoga's purpose is to free your body and mind. Therefore, we have no fixed rules on how to coordinate breath with movement, as is common in yoga and many schools of pelvic floor training. Most methods tense the pelvic floor during exhalation, and some recommend tensing during inhalation, but experts disagree on which is the best. Based on my experience with dance and bodywork systems like Feldenkrais and Linklater, I know that letting our breath come and go naturally enhances our freedom, expressiveness, and spontaneity.[52]

That's why we give ourselves the freedom to play with the breath here. This is an invitation to experiment with your breathing patterns and observe how your body responds.

In general, you'll observe that when you're breathing normally, your diaphragm will gently move your pelvic floor as described above. When you tense your pelvic floor while exhaling, this will feel very natural and strong. In contrast, if you tense your pelvic floor while inhaling, your pelvic floor will have to work harder against the pressure from your organs, and as a result, you'll be able to expand your rib cage and straighten out your entire posture more.

PRACTICE 10: Pelvic Floor Meditation

Once you've mastered pelvic floor breathing (Practice 9), I have a wonderful pelvic floor meditation for you. Let's try it now! Meditation trains your mind to focus and helps you recognize your true self. You will also see how meditation can help you have better sex in the chapter called "Really Good Sex."

1 Set your timer for five to twenty minutes.

2 Keeping your back straight, sit in the lotus position on the ground. If that's uncomfortable for you, choose a chair. Close your eyes. Your hands can rest loosely on top of each other in your lap with the tips of your thumbs touching—this centers you. If you rest them on your knees and turn your palms downward, your meditation will be grounding; with the palms up, it has an opening effect. Try all three positions to experience their effects for yourself, and use them as you need to, intuitively.

3 Close your eyes and bring your attention into your body. Observe where and how you're sitting, where your weight is, and how the ground feels.

4 Next, pay attention to your breath. Where can you feel it best? This could be in a different place every day. Now follow your breath down to the pelvic floor, and see if you can feel how it expands and contracts. Observe your breath in your pelvic floor.

5 Meditation is a mindfulness practice, among other things. In this meditation, you learn to focus your mind and to observe. This is not always easy, but it's worth it. The better you master your mind,

the easier it will be for you to do the pelvic floor practices effectively and the better you get to know yourself. You'll also love yourself more, but we'll get to that later.

If your attention wanders, if thoughts or memories come up, just acknowledge them and let them pass. This means you take notice of them, label them as "thinking," and place your attention back on your breath. For example, you might focus on inhaling and exhaling. Then a thought comes up: "My colleague is crazy." Note that you're thinking, and return to inhaling and exhaling. "What idiot drills holes into the wall at this hour?" Thinking. Back to inhaling. "Is this meditation already working?" Thinking. Back to exhaling...

What is important here is, first, that you put aside thoughts when you notice them, even if they seem incredibly interesting. Second, you don't get annoyed with yourself because you keep losing focus or follow your thoughts for minutes without even noticing. Be patient with yourself and return to the practice.

Our thoughts shape our brains; when you master your thoughts, you can consciously shape your brain. Furthermore, the more conscious you become of your thoughts, the more clearly you see that you are so much more than your thoughts. This will free you to be your true self. Remember, the journey is the destination. Your mindful awareness in any given moment is the goal. If you happen to experience deep insights and moments of oneness, those are a gift. Like orgasms, you can't force them, but you can make space and let them happen.

6 When your timer goes off, open your eyes. Notice how you feel, and enjoy the rest of your day with more confidence, radiance, and clarity.

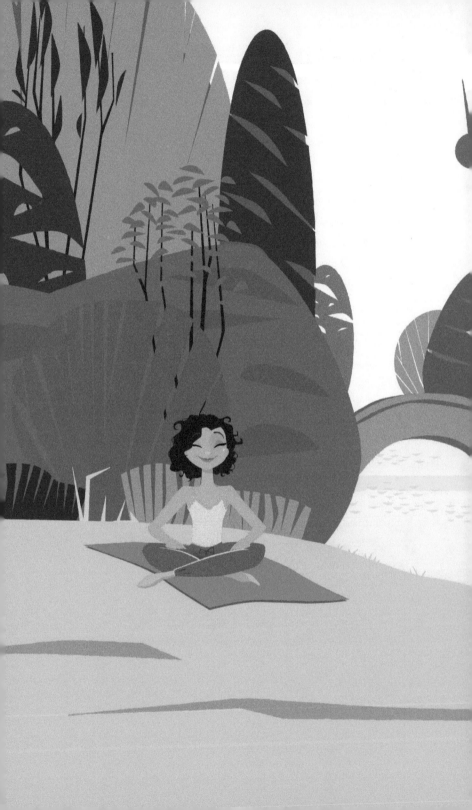

Try this meditation with your eyes open, too, so you get used to feeling your pelvic floor during your day.

The pelvic floor meditation helps you clear your mind like any other meditation, and in addition, it helps you to align your pelvic floor and feel incredibly radiant and sexy. In yoga, the pelvic floor is the seat of the root chakra. This chakra grounds us, giving us the feeling of being at home in ourselves and in this world.[53] Likewise, the Tao says the perineum contains an important energy center known as Huy Jin, which is the Gateway to Death and Life.[54] Better still, you don't need to believe in any of this for it to work. Just do the meditation and experience the effects for yourself.

Supple Hip Joints

Do you know where your hip joints are? Although they play an important role in our body's biomechanics, most people imagine them in the wrong place. Knowing and freeing your hip joints will not only improve the mobility of your pelvis, but it will also instantly give you a sexier walk and improve your posture.

PRACTICE 11: Locate and Mobilize the Hip Joints

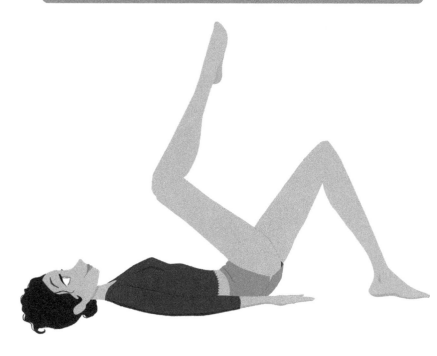

1 From the basic lying position, lift one of your legs and move it freely inside the hip joint. Try this with your leg straight and bent. Move your leg in all directions. The central point around which all movement revolves is your hip joint.

The head of your femur lies here in a joint socket shaped like a bowl called the acetabulum. It can be turned and rotated freely in all directions. The only other joint with this much mobility is the shoulder.

2   Put your leg back down and compare both sides. Do you notice a difference between your legs?

3   Repeat this game with the other leg.

4   Try this exercise standing as well, where you have more room to move your legs backward. Again, compare both sides.

This practice, done standing, is part of my daily warm-up. Try it out as a warm-up the next time you do sports or exercise.

Tip

Pelvic Floor Activation

In the following practices, we want to achieve a dynamic movement of the pelvic bones now that you know them. This is the most effective way to engage the levator ani, which, as we know, is the powerhouse of your pelvic floor. Once activated, we connect it with the surrounding muscles so it comes into its full power as the center of our musculoskeletal system. Owning your body like this, you'll feel more grounded and confident. Just make sure to keep your sphincter muscles, pussy, butt, and abs soft at all times (unless instructed otherwise). Consciously relax your whole pelvis in between.

PRACTICE 12: Pussy Cow

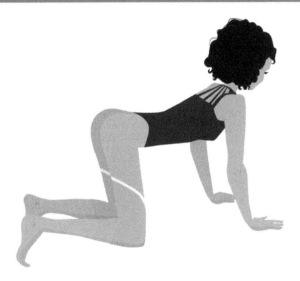

1 Start on your hands and knees, and let your spine hang downward just like an old cow. Your cervical spine is a natural extension of your spine here.

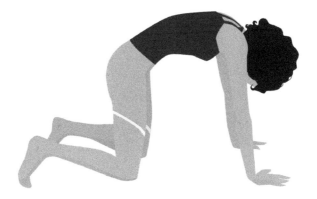

2 Now pull your belly button up toward the ceiling and round your
back like a cat. Let your head hang free.

3 Begin flowing between the two positions. Move back and forth
between them, observing the harmonious movement in your spine.
Try to loosen and mobilize all vertebrae evenly.

4 What is your pelvis doing? How are your pelvic bones moving? Try
to feel them in your body. Ideally, you would notice that, in the cow
position, your sit bones pull apart while your tailbone and sacrum
pull backward from the body and away from your pubic bone. This
makes your pelvis wider at the bottom, stretching your pelvic floor
wide open. Maybe you can feel a real pull in your first pelvic floor
layer? Try to relax there to give it a nice, natural stretch. In the cat
pose, the sit bones come together, and the tailbone and sacrum
approach the pubic bone again. This makes your pelvis narrower as
the pelvic floor contracts.

5 Now you can consciously draw your sit bones together in cat pose and notice the activation of your pelvic floor. Deliberately pull them apart in cow pose, and notice the stretch in your pelvic floor.

6 Next we will try this standing up. Set your legs apart a bit wider than the hips, placing your knees exactly above your feet. Rest your hands on your knees, so your butt moves backward. Do the cat and cow poses as described above.

7 To test the practice in this position, you can place your hands on your sit bones and feel the movement from the outside.

8 Then put one hand on your pubic bone, your fingers pointing down, and the other on the sacrum, with the fingers down as well. Try to feel the subtle nodding motion of the sacrum.

9 Slide your fingers further down your spine, so you can feel your tail-bone (coccyx). How is it moving? For most of us, it won't move on its own, but you can consciously wake it up. In cow pose, delibera-tely stretch your little tail away from your body as if you were trying to lift it up. Then let it go when you come into cat pose. Do you feel anything moving? Even if nothing moves, mentally include your tailbone in these movements from now on. Although our tailbone is an archaic part of our musculoskeletal system, it's nevertheless essential because it's connected with the whole pelvic floor.

10 While sitting or standing, feel how your breath widens the pelvic floor (Practice 9), and as it widens, actively move your little tail toward the back. This exercise helps you gradually return movement to your tailbone and dynamically trains your whole pelvic floor.

PRACTICE 13: Bring Your Sit Bones Together

1   In the basic lying position, place your feet in front of your pelvis. In this exercise, we don't move the pelvis. We let it stay on the floor and rest. All movement takes place inside the pelvis. Once again, feel your sit bones with your hands; then let go of the hands and sense your sit bones from the inside of your body. I Imagine a rubber band stretched between them that you can deliberately pull together. Bring the sit bones together and let go, together and let go—repeat those pulses while allowing your breath to flow calmly. Next, relax your pussy, the first layer of your pelvic floor, your butt, and your belly muscles. Take your time with this. Then let go and observe the effects in your body. Take a few breaths into your pelvic floor until it releases all tension.

2   Now pull your sit bones together, closer and closer, for as long as you can. Be sure to breathe calmly, and relax your first pelvic floor layer. Do this exercise for up to three minutes. Then relax for at least as long. Repeat the exercise one to three times, and then consciously let go.

3   Next we'll try some breathing patterns. Pull the sit bones together while you exhale. Observe your body. How does this interplay feel? Enjoy the fact that you're following the natural breathing pattern of the pelvic floor.

4   Now we'll do it the other way around. Pull your sit bones together while you inhale, and observe what happens in your body and in your whole ventral cavity. If you do this right, then inhaling and activating the pelvic floor will stretch your torso wide, a wonderfully uplifting and energizing feeling.

Contracting your sit bones as you inhale is a powerful activation for your pelvic floor, which can align your entire body. It's a wonderful practice to do anytime in your daily life. Afterward, it's essential to let go.

PRACTICE 14: Twist Your Hip Bones

1 In the basic lying position, place your feet in front of your pelvis. Let your sit bones sink into the earth without moving your pelvis. Now let's move one sit bone at a time, going from right to left and left to right. Do you feel how you can activate both sides of your pelvic floor independently of each other? This is important for an elegant walk.

2 Next, move your sit bones up and down. Imagine they're little feet that you swing as if you were trying to take big steps with them, and notice whether you can feel some movement in your sacroiliac joint. Relax and observe the effects on your pelvis and body.

3 Feel how both sides of your pelvis and your sacrum lie on the ground. Place your hands on your iliac bones and imagine how they rotate in opposite directions: one turns to the front and one to the back. Maybe you can already feel movement. You are moving your pelvis from your pelvic floor, which is the foundation for biomechanically sound walking.

4 Investigate how much movement you have in each joint between the sacrum and both of the hip bones. Are both sides equally flexible? Are they symmetrical?

If you notice your pelvis isn't symmetrical, don't worry too much about it. You'll be able to equalize both sides gradually with this gentle practice. Every irregularity in the pelvis has an effect on the whole body, which has adapted itself to this uneven position over years or decades. Notice how your body adjusts to this new information. Awareness, patience, and care will lead you to your best personal alignment, so don't try to force anything. That would only create resistance.

PRACTICE 15: Roll the Pelvis Up

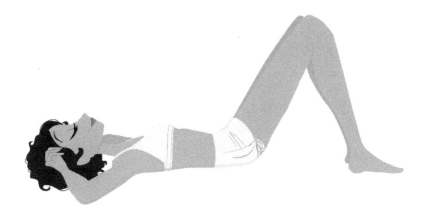

1 Start by relaxing in the basic lying position, and let your pelvis drop down toward the ground. Bring your sit bones together toward the perineum. Once you've moved them as far as you can, bring your tailbone toward your perineum as well. Then pull your tailbone and sit bones up toward your knees. Keep your belly completely relaxed so it's sinking toward the ground. Look for the first sign of tension, followed by a delicate movement in your pelvis. Repeat this a few times. Afterward, relax and let your pelvis drop down deep into the earth.

2 Bring the sit bones and tailbone once again toward the perineum, then up toward the knees. Now continue and observe how your pelvis slowly rolls up toward the ceiling. Before your pelvis leaves the floor, let it all roll back in the same way. Repeat this subtle yet powerful practice for as long as you wish. Always relax in between, lengthening your tailbone away from yourself.

3 Next, roll your pelvis in and out using the strength of your pelvic floor. When you roll the pelvis toward the back, let your back hollow. Observe how your pelvis moves your entire spine from head to toe.

4 Increase the speed until your entire body start to swing. This allows your spine to relax, soften, and realign. If you release a lot of tension in your body, you may find yourself laughing.

PRACTICE 16: The Tailbone as a Tail

1 Imagine the end of your spine curling up to the ceiling. Feel how this gradually builds up tension in the pelvic floor, as if it might roll up if your pelvis weren't so heavy.

2 What if your tailbone was a mighty tail like our ancestors used to have? Move your tailbone from left to right and pretend it's the powerful fin of a fish or the tail of a big, beautiful cat. Relax and feel the effects in your body.

3 Now imagine your tail is a rolled-up chameleon tail. Let it unroll down toward the earth until it lengthens on the ground. It will contract again by itself, and then you can let it stretch on the ground again. Relax everything. How does your body feel now?

4 Now draw circles with the tip of your little tail. Make them bigger, then smaller, and then change direction. After a few minutes, consciously let everything go.

5 Repeat all of the exercises playfully, this time with awareness of your whole spine, head, jaw, tongue, and eyes.

Do you notice anything moving in your face as well?
We are vertebrate animals. In the course of our evolution, we developed from the spine, and this is also how we develop as embryos in the womb to this day. The nerves and tissue of our face are deeply connected to our entire spine. That's one more reason why our spinal health affects all of our being.

During your day, keep playing with the idea of a cat's tail and think of yourself as a wild animal. This is not only fun, but it's also sexy, and it strengthens your instincts. Speaking coach KC Baker recommends this technique for public speaking. It also comes handy in meetings or when you're flirting.

Tip

PRACTICE 17: Chain Reaction

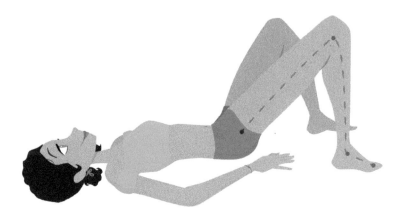

1 In the basic lying down position, press your right foot into the ground, and see if you notice a chain reaction through your ankle, knee, and hip joint to the pelvis and the pelvic floor. There is no movement visible from the outside; you can only feel it internally. Take your time to build the connections. Do you feel how your pelvic floor activates? Do you feel how your hip joint opens? Repeat this entire sequence a few times in slow motion. Then let go and observe your body. Do you notice a difference between your right and left hip joints and legs? Now changes sides.

2 Push your right foot firmly into the ground and observe how your pelvis begins to move slowly. Keep your knees pointing up toward the ceiling at all times. You can feel how your pelvis becomes lighter on the right side. Its center of gravity gradually moves to the left, twisting your pelvis to the side. Observe how this movement continues through your spine into your body. Do this exercise slowly a few times and then change sides.

3 Now alternate both sides and enjoy the gentle massage of your
sacrum.

4 Repeat the exercise a bit faster now until you build a loose swinging
movement. Play with the speed and size of the movement. What
feels best for your body today? Can you feel your sacroiliac joints
open?

5 Advanced version: You can refine this practice and make it more
effective by pressing not the whole foot into the ground but only
the metatarsophalangeal joint, which connects the big toe with the
ball of your foot. See if you can trigger the chain reaction from this
big toe joint. Stretch your legs out, relax, and observe the effects.

6 Leave the left leg lying on the ground while placing the right foot
back up like before. Extend your arms loosely on the floor next to
your head. Initiate the chain reaction with your right leg. The knee
stays pointing at the ceiling. Enjoy how far you can roll now and
how this movement flows through your body like a wave. Relax.
Change sides.

This practice is great for relaxing during your
day or if you have a backache (although you
will have fewer and fewer of those as you
improve your posture with Pussy Yoga).

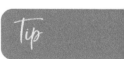

PRACTICE 18: Loosen Up—Shake Your Legs Toward the Sky

This practice is one that your body might intuitively crave between doing the other practices. From the basic lying position, lift your legs straight up and shake them vigorously. Kick your feet away from your body, either softly or with a lot of power and follow your flow. Allow the trembling to echo through your whole body and let it shake.

Tip

You can do this practice any time you like. Not only does it relax your pelvis and your legs, but it also helps the circulation in your pelvis and back—so it's grounding, loosening, and relaxing if you happen to have a backache or period pain.

Sensuous and Strong

In the following practices, tune into your sensuousness. Feel and enjoy your body, your energy, and your emotions. Feel your pussy; open your heart. Play with tension and with letting go. Dance with it and feel sexy.

PRACTICE 19: Inner Hip Circle—Lying Down

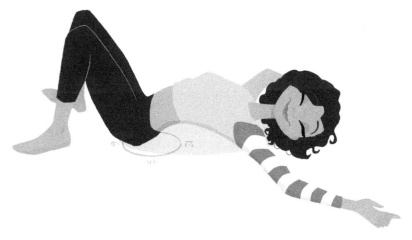

1 Start again in the basic lying down position and let your pelvis sink into the ground. Then rock it back and forth by alternating weight toward the lumbar spine (lower back) and the tailbone (as in Practice 15). Now rock your pelvis from right to left with your knees pointing upward (as in Practice 17). Once both movements are smooth, imagine your pelvis is on top of a clock. The upper part of your sacrum is at twelve o'clock, and your tailbone is at six o'clock, with your right hip joint at nine o'clock and your left at three o'clock.

2   Now roll your tailbone up so the upper part of your sacrum presses
    down on the twelve, and roll around until the right side is on
    the nine. Continue until your tailbone pushes down on six; then
    smoothly roll through three and twelve. Imagine every single hour
    on the clock and roll over each one as evenly as possible.

3   Make whole circles and let the pelvis sink heavily into the earth as
    you do so. Circle in both directions and investigate which direction
    and which part of the clock is particularly easy or particularly hard
    for you.

4   Feel how your pelvis moves your whole body as you circle and let go
    more and more. Let yourself be moved, take your arms with you,
    and enjoy your sensuousness.

PRACTICE 20: Inner Hip Circles on Your Belly

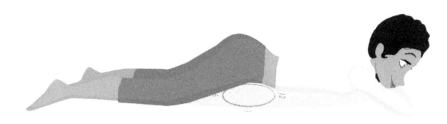

1   Lie on your belly. You can put your forehead on your hands so your
    spine is straight and relaxed. Imagine a clock under your pelvis (as
    in Practice 19).

2 Tilt your pelvis from six o'clock to twelve o'clock and back. Which muscles activate? Relax your pussy and your butt muscles, and try to move from the inside with your pelvic floor. Test out different ways of making it as easy, sensuous, and effective as possible. Play with the speed and size of the movement as well. This movement is essential for good sex, so dedicate a bit more time to it.

3 Now roll the pelvis from side to side and observe how you can make this movement both as efficient and as big as possible. Experiment and try to move from your pelvic floor. Rest whenever you need and feel the effects on your body.

4 Next, try making a sensuous and consistent pelvic circle while lying on your belly, slowly at first and then faster. Try out both directions.

5 Next, make this circle a full body experience. Move and stretch your body. Feel how gravity pulls you down and hugs your body to the earth.

PRACTICE 21: Enjoy Gravity and Levity

In our Pussy Yoga practice, we always work with gravity and use it as a way to consciously relax the body. For example, when we lie down and push a foot against the ground, we're consciously using the earth's gravity to pull the rest of the body down instead of pulling from both sides. This differentiated, almost lazy way of moving is more organic and effective than pushing yourself up by force and with tension. Watch big cats in nature, observe how they move with gravity, lie down, and get up again. All of it looks effortless and poised. Use this body knowledge not only for all of the practices here, but also during sex and when you roll over in bed or get up in the morning. Work with gravity, not against it.

1 Feel how the earth holds you, how gravity yearns for you. Feel how it pulls your body into the sheets or onto the ground. Feel your skin and your body. When you're sitting, feel how your butt and maybe your back and arms are held by gravity. This can be very sensuous and very relaxing.

2 Try it as well when you're walking. Feel how your legs move with gravity. Play with gravity as if it were a dance partner pulling your legs toward itself. Stay consciously in contact when you lift your legs.

3 Feel how your hand resists gravity and lifts above your head, then touches your hair from above or comes to rest on your cheek. Become aware of gravity as you let your hand glide down your face, your neck, and your breasts to your belly. Your senses and awareness are fully switched on.

4 Now lift your breasts consciously against gravity and move them in sensuous circles. You can also imagine a counterpart to gravity called "levity," which makes it easy for you to stand or sit tall with ease and grace.

5 Imagine that your tailbone is attached to the earth, and the rest of your body is hanging up from it. Feel how easily your body now orients itself upward.

6 Play with the idea that your feet are in magnetic shoes that pull you toward the ground. The rest of your body is falling away from the earth toward the universe.

PRACTICE 22: Pearl Necklace

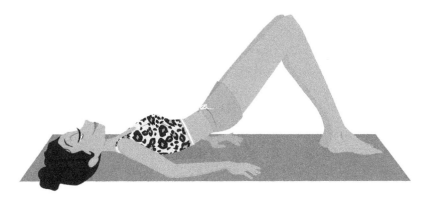

1 In the basic lying down position, place your feet hip-width apart again and start rocking your pelvis back and forth (as in Practice 15). Observe which muscles activate.

2 Starting from the tailbone, roll your pelvis upward, vertebra by vertebra, trying to move each vertebra individually. On the way up, carefully pull your pelvis up in slow motion, letting the spine lie heavy on the ground for as long as possible. Once you've reached your maximum height, keep your pelvis up while, again in slow motion, you roll your spine down, vertebra by vertebra. The pelvis slowly follows the spine, which becomes more and more supple.

3 You can imagine your body as a necklace of big marble beads lying at the bottom of the ocean. Pretend they're being slowly pulled upward by a fishhook attached to the lower end of your spine. One vertebra leaves the ground at a time and pulls the next vertebra with it, so there is more space between them for the intervertebral discs. On the way down, the thoracic vertebrae are the first to come

down while the pelvis stays up, still hanging on the hook. Roll down one after the other until the pelvis is once again heavy on the ground. Do this exercise at least three times in slow motion and then relax.

Tip

This practice will massage and strengthen your entire spine. Your body will love it if you do it every day. You can do it, for example, in bed in the morning.

PRACTICE 23: Hip Twist—Lying Down

1 Start in the basic lying position with your feet on the ground. Lift your pelvis to a comfortable height; then alternate pushing the right and left hip up. A loose twist starts to happen. Do this exercise slowly and then speed it up. Play with it.

2 Become aware of the chain reaction from your foot to your knee to your hip and your pelvic floor. Let the pelvis relax without activating your butt. Roll down gently and relax.

PRACTICE 24: Figure Eight—Lying Down

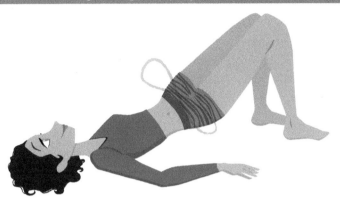

1 Start again in the basic lying position with your feet on the ground. Lift your pelvis to a comfortable height and draw a figure eight with your hip. As in the twist, bring your right hip bone up and then push the whole pelvis slightly to the right. Then twist your hips so your left hip bone comes up and moves to the left. Notice the chain reaction from your foot to your knee to your hip and to your pelvic floor. Relax while doing this exercise. It's intended to mobilize your hip joints and spine. Roll down gently and enjoy the feeling in your body.

2 Again, bring your hips up, and try to draw a figure eight in the other direction, bringing your right hip bone up. Then push your whole pelvis slightly to the left. Next twist your hips so your left hip bone comes up and moves to the right. Play with the speed and keep changing direction. See what feels really good to you.

This is one of the movements I do every morning in bed to loosen and stretch everything before I get up. It's so delicious!

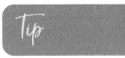

PRACTICE 25: Big Hip Circles—Lying Down

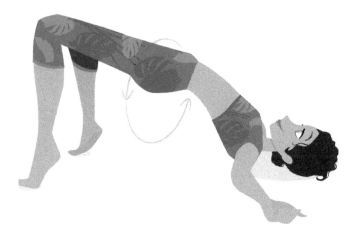

1　From the basic lying position, bring your pelvis up, easy and relaxed, with the spine keeping its natural S-curve. Then bring your pelvis as far as you can to the side, then down and to the left. Slowly move in huge enjoyable circles. Inhale when you lift your pelvis, and exhale with pleasure when you lower it back down.

2　Try this practice on tiptoes, and let your arms move sensuously on the ground or over your body, just as your body likes it. Make it a sensuous dance.

3　Try making sounds as you exhale. Say, "Aahhh," "Oohhh," "Mmmh," "Shhh," or just make the noises your body wants to make. According to the teachings of the Tao, these sounds dissolve blocks and improve your energy flow. Try it. Your body will love it!

PRACTICE 26: Move the Legs from the Pelvic Floor

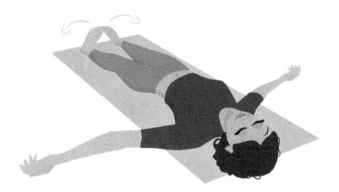

1 Lie down with your legs stretched out hip distance apart and your toes pointing toward the ceiling. Now turn your legs from the hip joint so your feet point inward and outward in turn. Feel how your femurs turn in your hip joints.

2 Now observe what's moving in your pelvic floor and around your pussy. Try to do this practice from your pelvic floor. Feel your levator ani in its entirety; see how it activates at the back when you turn your legs out and on the sides when it turns your legs in. Observe what's happening in your sacroiliac joints as well.

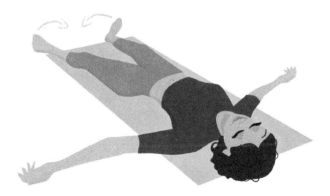

3 Turn both feet to the right and the left at the same time and observe your internal muscles moving. Relax.

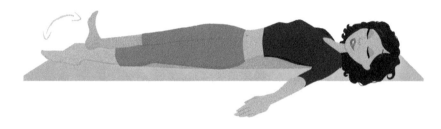

4 In the same starting position, flex your feet by pulling your toes toward yourself and then point them away from your body like a ballerina. What's your pelvis doing now? Can you control this movement from your pelvic floor?

5 Now flex the right foot and point the left. Alternate the foot positions and observe how your pelvic floor works.

6 Next push the right heel away from your pelvis, then the left, working purely with the strength of your pelvic floor. This helps you feel how you can activate your pelvic floor while walking.

7 Now let's get up and try this out, taking one step at a time. Push your big toe joint firmly into the ground when you push yourself forward. What effect does this have on your walk?

 You can also feel the effects while you drive a car, specifically when you accelerate, break, or change gears. But please keep your eye on the road!

PRACTICE 27: Pelvic massage—Open All Pelvic Joints

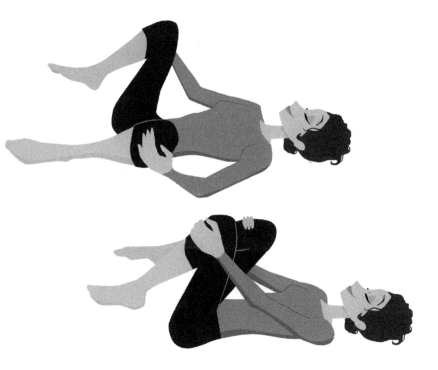

1 Lie on your back, pull your knees toward yourself, and place your hands on your knees. Keep them loosely together and move them from side to side. Feel how your femurs move in the hip joints and whether anything moves in your sacroiliac joints between the hip bones and the sacrum.

2 Now bring your knees apart and back together again. Investigate how your body moves on the inside. Then move them forward and backward one by one.

This practice is really great for relaxing
before you go to sleep.

3 Next bring your knees together, and let them circle above your hip
while they remain connected.

4 Try circling them in opposite directions by first holding both knees
together. Then bring one close to your chest and one away from
your chest. Next, move them apart to each side. Finally, move the
leg that is closer to your torso away from you and pull the other
toward you so you have two circles running in opposite directions.

5 Then take hold of your feet from the side or from the top over your
toes, and bring the knees to the right and left of your belly toward
the floor like babies do. Relax in this position and let your pelvis
drop down deeper and deeper with every breath.

6 From this baby position, use your arms to control your legs and
feet so you can roll your body from side to side. Try not to use
momentum, but instead do it in slow motion and work with
gravity. Use this practice to open all of the joints in your pelvis,
stretching all muscles, tendons, and ligaments.

7 In the same position, your hands still on your feet, stretch your
feet away from your body as far as possible and explore your options here. How can you move your legs? What feels good? Where
would you like more suppleness?

PRACTICE 28: Pelvic Clock—Standing Up

I used to do this exercise backstage right before every show to ground myself and become more present. It works like a charm!

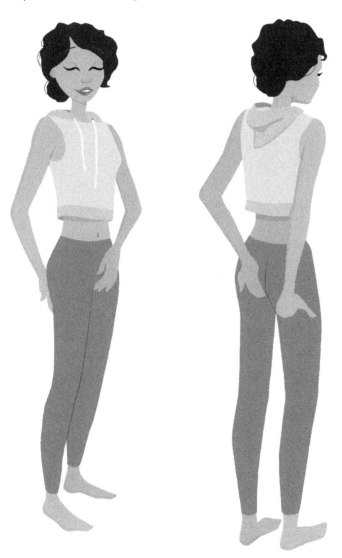

1   While standing up, touch the four lower points on your pelvis (sit bones, pubic bones in front, and tailbone at the back). Visualize the pelvic floor between all four points. For this practice, you can imagine your pelvic floor like a clock with its quarters. Twelve o'clock is on the pubic bones, and six o'clock is on the tailbone. Three o'clock is on the right sit bone, nine o'clock on the left. Now place a finger from your left hand on the right pubic bone and a finger from your right hand on your right sit bone. Massage both points to anchor them more deeply in your body awareness. Between these two points is the front right quadrant of your pelvic clock: twelve to three. Feel into it and imagine this exact place in your body. Notice how it expands and contracts as you breathe.

2   Do this exercise for at least ten relaxed breaths. Drop your hands and feel into your body. What has changed in your body and in your perception? Walk a few steps to observe the difference in your mobility and your connection with the earth.

3   Then place a finger from your left hand on the tailbone and a finger from your right hand on your right sit bone. Massage both points. Between them is the back right quadrant of your pelvic clock: three to six. Feel into it and imagine this exact place in your body. Notice how it expands and contracts as you breathe. Do this exercise for another ten breaths. Then drop your hands and observe. What has changed now? How do both sides of your body feel? I hope you notice a big difference in mobility on the right side of your body and in how grounded you feel.

4   Repeat the practice on the left side of your body as well.

Do this practice when you want excellent posture and performance. It instantly creates a more relaxed and powerful presence.

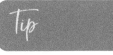

PRACTICE 29: Feeling Is Sexy

You already know how effective it is to practice sensing your body. Take the time between the exercises and after your Pussy Yoga practice to walk around the room and observe the sensations in your body. How does your walk feel now? How does your posture feel? How do you perceive your environment? You are probably much more present now, see things more sharply, and feel lighter, both physically and emotionally. However you feel and whatever you notice will be completely different each time. The goal of this exercise is not to attain a certain state but to practice conscious observation and integration.

Bring this sensing practice into your daily life. Sense yourself when you're waiting for the coffee dispenser or at a red light—feel how you're standing and feel your pelvic floor. Observe what's going on in your body when you're walking and climbing stairs. When you're dancing at a party, feel how you're moving. Conscious sensuous movement is always sexy. It's what made my shows magnetic. Your audience always feels what you feel. Being conscious in your body is sexy and radiates confidence; it is never sleazy or needy. Try it out the next time you want to feel seductive!

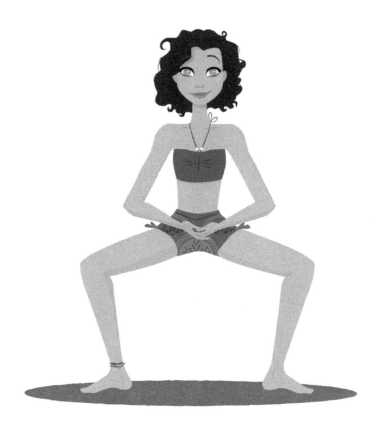

PRACTICE 30: Pelvic Floor in Plié

1 Place your feet a little wider than hip-width apart, the toes pointing slightly to the side, and let your pelvis drop into a plié, which is a shallow squat that leaves your heels on the ground. Your knees should always be aligned over your toes, not collapsing inward or outward. Move your pelvis up and down a few times in this position.

2 Feel how your pelvis moves on the inside. You can use your hands to see if you can observe any movement in your bones. If you pay

attention, you will notice that the sit bones move apart as you go down and the iliac crests move toward each other at the top. Coming back up has the opposite effect. Try to make this micro-movement bigger in your mind.

3 Now imagine how your pelvic floor contracts as you come up, and when you go down, consciously push your tailbone toward the back. Feel the stretch in your pelvic floor.

Pelvic Floor and Dancing

When I started integrating my pelvic floor into my dancing, it dramatically improved my performance. This integration also made the pelvic floor training so much more effective and fun. I called what I had discovered the "Essence of Bellydance," as it was the essence that I had been looking for on my quest to find the key to great dancing. Practicing this Essence of Bellydance in turn helped me and my students get closer to our very own personal essence.

In Essence of Bellydance, we combine the sensual art of Bellydance with Pelvic Floor Integration and contemporary awareness techniques. Our practice connects us to our body wisdom and our intuition. It also makes us stronger, enhances our orgasms, and makes our births and recoveries easier.

In one way or another, this essential feminine way of moving has been handed down from woman to woman over thousands of years in various archaic dances. This ancient knowledge has been lost to us through our patriarchal civilization and our disconnected nuclear families (e.g., outsourcing gynecology to doctors and hospital births). But now we can rediscover it and share it with each other—our body shows us the way.

If you want to learn these movements and many more with me, I recommend my free online course on EssenceBellydance.com.
If you want to go even deeper, join me in my Sensuous Dance Lifestyle Program at SensuousWorkout.com, where I introduce you to my signature pelvic floor practice and sensuous dance.
Our international team and I would also love to guide you personally in one of our workshops or maybe in the Essence of Bellydance™ teacher training. You can find our teacher directory and a calendar of events on EssenceBellydance.com.

Below, I've selected the most effective movements from the Essence of Bellydance™ method for you. These movements train your pelvic floor efficiently and integrate it into your natural flow of movement. They also enable you to move better in your everyday life, and of course when you're having sex.

You can dance in front of a mirror if you wish. No matter where you are, close your eyes every now and then to feel the movement better from the inside and to feel the sensuous pleasure rising in your body. Our basic position is standing upright with the knees slightly bent. The feet are placed directly below your hip joints, and for the basic exercises here, they point to the front. Your pelvis and your head should feel free, and your spine should remain upright and long at all times.

Soon, you will notice how these dance movements switch on naturally, both on the dance floor and in your sex life. But this isn't just a technique. When you dance like this and connect with your pelvis, you'll get to know other sides of yourself that you may not have noticed before. It's also possible that stuck emotions will begin to move and old blocks dissolve.

Experiencing your dancing body will inevitably make you feel beautiful and sexy, and that will free you up for even better sex.

Don't worry if the movements feel stiff at the beginning or if they look awkward. Explore the movements in your body with playfulness and curiosity. That's the best way to master them. Don't cheat and stay in your old familiar movement patterns. Instead allow yourself to tune into your feminine sensuousness and feel the quality of your movement.

To make it more fun, pick music that inspires you to dance. If you get swept up, forget the exercises and just dance. You can continue with the practice later on. Dancing freely is not only fun, but it also mobilizes your body and gives you access to your Felt Sense and your wild feminine intuition. Feel yourself and your energy from the inside and enjoy living in your wonderful, miraculous body.

PRACTICE 31: Hip Tilt

1 From the basic standing position, tilt your pelvis slowly forward and backward (as in Practice 15) and observe which parts of your body you use to create this movement. What's happening in your hip joints and your spine? Try to relax your upper body, and keep it still so your pelvis only moves below your belly button.

2 Once the Hip Tilt feels good in your body, focus on the movement of your sit bones, which are moving forward and backward with your pelvis. If you observe carefully, you will notice that they also move toward each other as they come forward and away from each other as they go backward. Activate your pelvic floor by consciously moving them together as you bring them toward the front; then let go and observe them moving apart again.

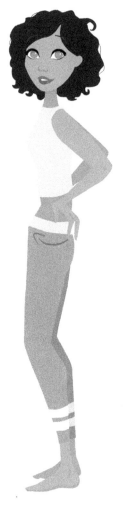

3 Do the movement with the pelvic floor activation slowly at first, then like an easy thrusting, and then faster until it's a controlled trembling. Let the movement flow and try to relax as much as possible.

4 Now back to tilting in slow motion. Place your attention on your tailbone at the lower end of your spine. Mentally attach a golden thread there and pull it through your legs to the front when you bring your sit bones to the front. Let your tailbone swing back when you bring your sit bones to the back.

5 Next, imagine extending your tailbone into a beautiful animal tail of your choosing, maybe a lioness. Let it swing back and forth elegantly while you tilt your pelvis.

6 Place one hand on your sacrum, the part of your spine between your two hip bones, and observe whether you notice a slight nodding and a movement between the sacrum and the hip bones. Don't worry if you can't feel anything at the beginning; it will all come in time.

7 Can you sense around which point in your pelvis the whole movement rotates? It's the center of your pelvis.

PRACTICE 32: Hip Seesaw

1 From the standing position, distribute your weight evenly over both feet, and maintain this distribution during the exercise. Keep your knees slightly bent. Now bend your right knee more while keeping your left knee where it is. Then swap the knees and keep alternating so an easy rocking or seesaw motion starts to happen in your hips. When you bend your left knee, your right hip comes up, and when you bend your right knee, your left hip comes up. Your upper body does not engage in the movement. Just let it float above your pelvis.

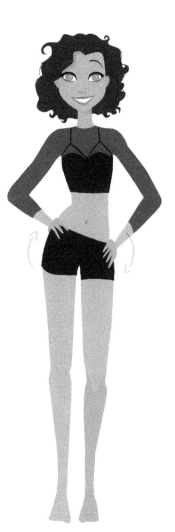

2 Where is the center of this movement? Around which point does it revolve? It's the center of your pelvis, which, according to yoga, houses your sexual chakra.

3 Now envision your tailbone swinging from side to side like a tail.

4 If this seesaw begins to feel easy, speed it up and play with the tempo. It's fun with some rhythmic music. Maintain full control of the movement so it matches the rhythm of the music.

5 Now make it faster and faster, observing how your pelvis, your thighs, your butt, and your belly begin to shake and vibrate. Speed it up even more until you lose control and the shaking takes over. Let everything shake: your thighs, your butt, your belly. Play with this movement for as long as you like. Keep your breathing relaxed and feel the energies that your body releases. If you get stuck, just go back to the beginning and slowly build the movement up again. Like relaxation and ecstasy, this movement cannot be forced; it can only be allowed, like orgasms.

Tip Done quickly, this movement is used in many ancient cultures to reach ecstasy or let go of trauma. It helps the pelvis and the entire body relax. Try letting go more and more. This loose shaking is called a "shimmy" in belly dance. It's something only a few women find easy to do, but in surveys, it's always the most popular belly dance move.

PRACTICE 33: Inner Hip Circle

If we now combine Hip Tilts and Seesaws, we get a movement called the Inner Hip Circle or Afro. This movement exists in cultures all over the world, and its character is always sexual. The movement has four stages connected to a grinding rotation. You rotate around the center point of your pelvis.

This practice is essential for good sex and is a wonderful way to train your pelvic floor by dancing. You can do it every day. Just put on some music and go.

1 Let your right hip come up, like in the Seesaw; then tilt your pelvis forward so the sit bones come together and your pelvic floor activates. Now bring your left hip up and let everything relax. Connect all four stages of movement to a circle that is centered in the middle of your pelvis.

2 Dance this Hip Circle in all of the variations you can imagine. Focus on the center of your pelvis and give in to your passion and flow.

PRACTICE 34: Side Slide with Chain Reaction

1 From the basic standing position, slightly bend your knees and slide your hip softly from side to side. Don't let your upper body join the movement. If you look down your body, your breasts should stay over your feet as you slide your hips from side to side.

2 Pay attention to keeping your hip bones at the same level, parallel to the ground and parallel to the front. This gets easier if you actively include your knees in the movement. As you slide your hips to the right, bend your right leg at the same time. This allows you to balance out the hip. Do the same thing on the other side. This move isn't easy and requires a lot of coordination in the beginning, but like all movements that we struggle to coordinate at first, it's a great workout for your brain as well.

3 Now we add in the pelvic floor activation. Notice how, when you slide your hip, you also shift your weight in the same direction. This means that in one moment, your right foot bears more weight and pushes into the ground more, and the next moment, it's your left foot. To focus on training the pelvic floor, we increase the pressure.

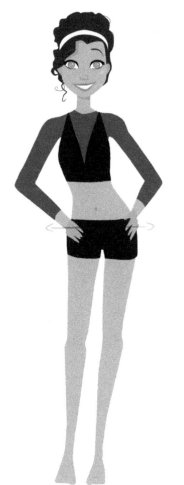

Push your right foot into the ground as you slide your hip to the right. Feel the chain reaction (as in Practice 17) from your foot to your ankle, then into the knee, the hip joint, and to the right side of the pelvic floor. As you've already experienced, you can control both sides individually.

4 Once you get this chain reaction, imagine you're pushing into the ground from your pelvic floor. Push so hard that the other foot could easily lift off the ground. Now you can start walking with this movement.

5 Try to push your big toe joint into the floor and build a more refined chain reaction from here.

This trains your pelvic floor to activate with every step. You don't even need the hip slide anymore. As you walk around during your day, see if you can feel how your pelvic floor automatically activates.

PRACTICE 35: Hip Twist

1 Without moving your upper body, bring your right hip bone to the front and then the left, creating a loose twisting motion. Do it from the center of your pelvis, softly and very precisely. Twist as far as you can without moving your upper body or your arms. If you look down your body, your breasts should be exactly above your feet and should not move. Only the hips twist.

2 Feel how you twist around the center of your pelvis. Play with the tempo and speed it up until your pelvis shakes around your center.

3 Once you've perfected this, shift your weight and twist in your right hip joint, then the left. Do it slow and fast, and enjoy it.

PRACTICE 36: Double Cone for a Sexy Walk

Now we combine the Hip Twist with the Hip Seesaw to a Double Cone. This doesn't sound very sexy, but it will give you a sexy walk that also trains your pelvic floor.

1 Seesaw your right hip bone up and then twist it backward. Let it come down and twist it to the front. The other hip bone is doing the same movement, so you stay centered. Keep doing these movements until they flow smoothly, which might take a while. Feel the point in your pelvis around which the whole movement revolves. It's like in the Hip Circle, the Twist, the Seesaw, and the Tilt—exactly at the center of your pelvis.

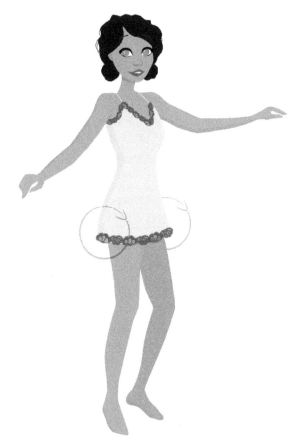

2 Next, we turn the whole thing around. Seesaw your right hip bone up and then twist it forward. Let it come down and twist it to the back. Keep doing these movements until they flow smoothly. Be easy on yourself, smoothing this out might take a while.

 As you walk around during the day, try to take the idea of this movement with you. Feel the center of your pelvis and notice how your hip bones circle easily backward around this point. This will give your gait majesty and suppleness.

PRACTICE 37: Big Hip Circle

This Big Circle mobilizes your hip joints and all of the joints in your pelvis. It trains and stretches the pelvic floor dynamically. This is also one of the practices that I never miss in my daily warm-up.

1 Place your feet a little wider than shoulder-width apart. Then push your pelvis as far as possible to the front, then to the side and the back. Here, I mean really far back so your sit bones stretch toward the back wall. Then you move on to the other side and again to the front. Connect those points in a smooth large circle with your pelvis. Draw this circle nice and wide, making it bigger each time, as if you were trying to touch all of the walls in the room with your hips. Once you're satisfied, try it in the other direction and see whether this side feels any different.

2 Now let's add the pelvic floor. Observe how your pelvic bones are moving inside your body. While you push your pelvis to the front, your sit bones come together, and you can consciously activate your pelvic floor here by pulling them even closer together. Then let go gradually as you move to the side. Observe how your sit bones and your pelvic floor slowly widen. When your pelvis has reached the maximum extension at the back with your butt sticking out as far as possible, consciously open your sit bones wider, and stretch your tailbone away from the pubic bone. This gives your pelvic floor a really nice active stretch.

3 You can bend your knees slightly or straighten your legs. Try out which feels better for you. The aim of the backward movement is also to stretch the backs of the thighs (the hamstrings), so keep your lower back either straight or slightly hollow.

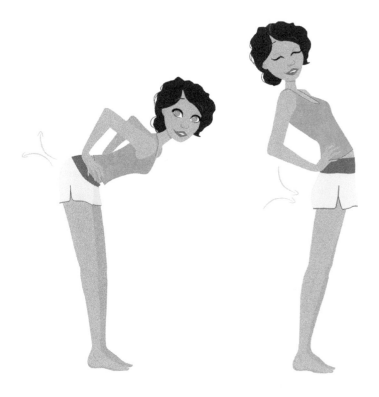

4 Observe the movement in your hip joints and feel how it frees them.

5 To make it more fun, you can involve your entire body. Once your
   pelvis is at the back, you can drop your spine down, and let your
   head sink toward the ground, so it gets included in the rotation as
   well. Use the weight of your hair (if yours is long).

6 To kick it up a notch: As you push your pelvis to the front, the
   movement becomes even more intense if you stretch your head back
   as an extension of your spine, long and elegant. Let your hips guide
   your movement and enjoy the ride.

PRACTICE 38: Free Dance

Find some music that makes you want to dance and do a free, wild, and vulnerable dance just for you. With or without a mirror, dressed or naked, let your body dance and enjoy the adventure. This is your time to express and explore all sides of yourself. I have my best ideas when I dance, and I can say that dance literally saved my life many times. Most women who give it a serious try report similar experiences.

Here are some ideas for bringing more dance into your life:

★ Notice every time your body wants to move throughout the day and use it. If you hear good music, your hips will probably want to move. If you feel tense after a meeting, your body would probably love to shake it out. I don't know anyone who dances too much.

★ Dance to a song after your Pussy Yoga session or any other workout.

★ Dance to one song every morning.

★ Take dance breaks during your day, and dance through your office or your home. If your work environment doesn't allow it, at least do some Hip Circles or shimmies every time you use the bathroom.

★ If your intuition reminds you of a song, find it and let yourself be moved. My intuition always gives me what I need in that moment. I trust it even if it seems totally ridiculous. Sometimes I listen to it over and over again on repeat, or I let the algorithm of the streaming service present me with other suggestions, which are usually perfect as well.

★ If you feel unsatisfied or you're plagued with negative emotions or worries, don't push them away. You can loosen them up or process them wonderfully by dancing. Pick a track spontaneously as guided by your intuition, or dance without music. Move through your emotions. Let your feelings flow through you and watch them shift. Stay open, free of judgments and expectations. You can combine this later with the Emotional Freedom practice (see the "Really Good Sex" chapter).

Mirror Mirror—From Object to Being

Because we have such wonderful minds, it's perfectly normal to be outside of our body every now and then when we make plans, read, watch films, remember beautiful times, or are completely absorbed in contemplation or work.

Looking at our bodies in the mirror is another habit that brings us out of the body. I observed this as a dancer. While I was training, I realized I wasn't in my body, but I was watching a body in the mirror, which I steered with a remote control, so to speak. I used my body as a 3D puppet to achieve the esthetic effects that I imagined. I paused, stepped in front of the mirror, and looked at my body. I saw this being coming toward me and at the same time tried to be present in my body—a fascinating game with consciousness. Try it sometime. Are you the observer or the observed?

We unfold our true presence and power only when we are in our body with our full consciousness, when we live from within. If we watch our body from the outside, we alienate ourselves from it. We turn it into an object and evaluate it from the outside, usually in a less-than-friendly manner. However, we move toward unconditional self-love when we learn to feel our body from the inside and experience it as the wonderful organism that it is.

I therefore that recommend you remain fully present with all of your senses in every physical activity, not just during Pussy Yoga. Try not listening to podcasts while you run and not watching videos in the gym. Instead, dive into your body completely. This not only trains your sensuous skills but also allows you to reap greater results from your workout.

Pelvic Floor Training in the Office

The following practices are suitable for the office because we can do almost all of them right at our desk without drawing attention, or we can do them out and about during the day. You will see the best results if you have mastered them beforehand as part of your Pussy Yoga training at home.

PRACTICE 39: Mentally Align Your Pelvis

The following practice is done only in the mind, without consciously moving any body parts. Little by little, it becomes so powerful that it activates the right muscles to align your pelvis perfectly.

1 Whether lying, sitting, or standing, imagine that your pubic bones are pulling up toward your belly button.

2 Now imagine that your tailbone is pulling down to the ground. How does this dynamic feel in your pelvis? How does the rest of your body react? Feel free to spend five minutes on this exercise. It's a good investment.

You can do this exercise at your desk or while you're walking down the street. It will help you align your pelvis.

Tip

PRACTICE 40: Miniskirt—Balance Out Pelvic Tension

Like Practice 39, this exercise can be done in any position you can think of because you're working solely with your mind.

1 Imagine you're wearing a very short miniskirt, which is becoming tighter and tighter at the front of your pelvis and widening at the back. Follow this imagined movement mentally: in front, the fabric constantly pulls tighter, and at the back, it constantly stretches.

2 Observe how muscles activate deep in your pelvis and belly and how the backs of your hips and your lower back can relax, freeing your sacroiliac joints and hip joints. It's important that you do not tense a single muscle. It's purely your imagination that brings a tense pelvis and lower spine back into healthy balance and enables new neural connections, which are important for healthy alignment and pelvic floor toning.

Observe and see if you can notice the new alignment in your body.

This practice gives you great posture anywhere and anytime: in the elevator, at the traffic lights, or standing in line in the supermarket. I find it works best on chairs, for example, when sitting at your desk.

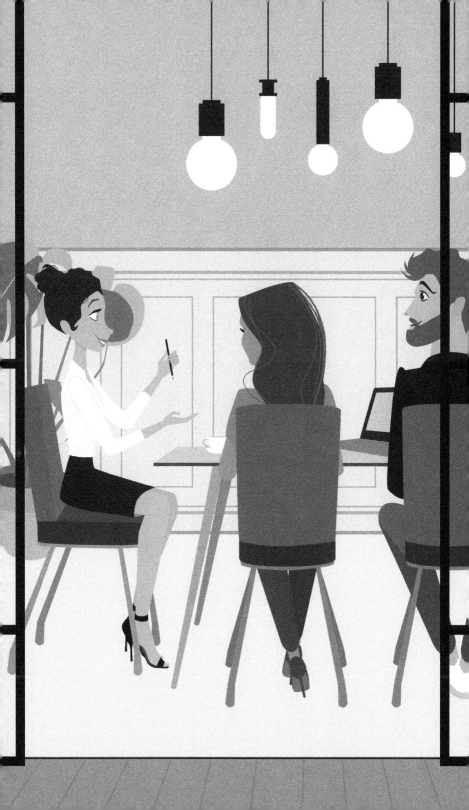

PRACTICE 41: Push Your Feet into the Ground

1 This is our basic sitting position. Sit on the edge of a chair, your feet about hip-width apart, placed flat and relaxed on the ground. You can do all of the sitting practices in high heels as well—just build a strong connection to the floor. Feel your sit bones. Let them drop deep into the seat beneath you. Align your spine by imagining every single vertebra and your head floating up to the ceiling.

2 Now push your right foot into the ground until you experience the chain reaction (as described in Practices 17 and 34) and feel the power building in your pelvic floor. Let go and change sides. Now alternate between the two sides and observe how the exercise affects the rest of your body. Practice with maximum intensity while keeping it as light and effortless as possible.

3 Play with the pressure and tempo. Feel whether both sides are symmetrical and how the chain reaction works through your whole body, helping you to align yourself perfectly.

4 If your upper body wants to turn, let it.

Stand up in between to analyze the effect on your posture. If your torso feels longer and more upright, you have done it perfectly.

5 If you feel like the foot with no weight on it wants to lift from the ground, let it come up a little. This creates the same dynamics as in walking—it's the perfect training and a wonderful integration for the pelvic floor!

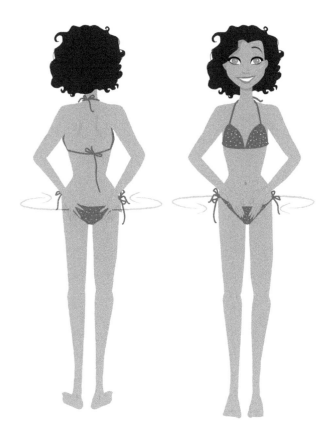

6 Now try to push both feet into the ground. Experiment again with pressure and speed, and observe what happens in your pelvic floor and your body.

7 If you notice that your levator ani activates and both sit bones come together, you're doing it right. Once your hips widen at the back and your lower abdominal muscles activate, you've mastered the pelvic floor integration, but make sure your first pelvic floor layer is relaxed.

PRACTICE 42: Push Your Knees Together and Apart

1 From our upright seated position: Place your hands on the inside of your knees or use something like a yoga block to keep them about four inches apart. Now push your knees together using the strength of your pelvic floor. Push against the resistance of your hands or the object. Nudge the block a few times, quickly and softly. Then increase the intensity until you reach your personal limit.

2 If you're using your hands for resistance, make sure your body posture is good so this exercise trains your whole body. Vary the position of your hands. Place them sometimes on the knee on the same side, sometimes crossing over. Let your breath flow easily.

3 Now push both of your sit bones into the seat at the same time.

4 Stand up and walk around the room as you observe your body.

5 Then do the same exercise, but pull your knees apart against the resistance from your hands. For extra support, you can tie a scarf or a strap around your thighs near the knees.

Tip

Most of these practices are very subtle. You can do them anywhere and anytime, whether you're sitting, standing, or lying down. Nobody will notice.

PRACTICE 43: Move Your Hip Bones in Opposite Directions

1 Sit on the edge of a chair and feel your sit bones. Let them drop deep into the seat beneath you.

2 Without moving your pelvis on the outside, move your sit bones in opposite directions, alternating forward and backward. Observe how your pelvic floor activates and connects with the muscles in your upper body. Which other muscles can you feel? Don't activate them deliberately. Focus only on the movement of your pelvic bones.

3 Now alternate pushing the sit bones into the seat, left and right. Observe how the different sides of your pelvic floor activate. Do both sides feel the same?

4 Next, imagine your sit bones are hanging in the air and alternate swinging them back and forth. Your hip bones will twist against each other as you do so. Can you feel a movement in your sacroiliac joints? Do you notice a difference between the sides? Try to let both sides swing with equal strength and ease. Observe.

5 Imagine your sit bones hanging in the air again, and lightly swing your sit bones together. Then let go, again and again, as if they could bounce together. Play with the tempo and your breath. Take some time to observe the effects on your body.

6 Lightly bring both sit bones together to the front, as if you were trying to move the seat of your chair forward with the power of your pelvic floor.

7 Let the sit bones sink into the seat again. Now pull back with your tailbone, as if you wanted to swing your tail backward. As you do so, feel into your pelvic floor, your sacrum, your sacroiliac joints, and your whole body. Repeat as often as you like; then relax your pelvic floor consciously.

PRACTICE 44: Riding a Chair

This one's funny, and it's a really effective practice for training your pelvic floor. Everything that we've learned so far flows into this practice. At the same time, you can increase your stamina for sex.

1 Sit astride on a chair with a soft cushion underneath if possible. Then ride the chair, letting your spine move as well.

2 Place both feet under your knees or further back if needed. Experiment with different positions. Now try moving the chair forward with the help of your pelvic floor. You will notice immediately how your pelvic floor activates powerfully. Enjoy the movement and feel the strength of your pelvic floor and its connection to the entire muscle system at your core.

3 Breathe easily and consciously, and relax your butt. As you thrust forward, actively push your sit bones toward the front and together, and then deliberately let them go. Make sure you're loose.

4 Get up and walk around to observe the effect of the practice.

5 Next time you ride, let your whole body take part. Throw your arms in the air and have fun!

This practice is very powerful, and
if you've done the other exercises
diligently, it activates your pelvic floor
in a wonderful way. It effectively
strengthens its connection
with the rest of your
body. But it's also just a
lot of fun, so do it any
time you feel stuck
and want to loosen
up. If you're on your
own, you can also
do it at your desk
while you work.

Tip

PRACTICE 45: Hanging and Breathing

Tip

This practice is great for a quick relaxing break in your day, especially if you have a sore back from standing or walking for a long time. If your legs are too tired, you can also do this exercise as a pure breathing practice while lying down. That makes it less effective, but it will still be fantastic.

1 Stand up comfortably and, starting from your head, gently bend forward, letting your spine roll down slowly. Try to feel every single vertebra move and loosen each as you do so. Once you've reached the bottom, just hang for a bit. Find a comfortable position for your arms, either resting on the ground or folded.

2 Now feel your breath. Notice it without changing it. Just observe. Where do you notice it first? Try feeling it on the tip of your nose, then inside your nose. Can you also feel your sinuses? Next follow it down your throat, your windpipe, and your lungs. Where do your lungs take up space?

3 Now feel how your breath expands your ribcage. Where can you feel your ribs? Where does your ribcage widen? For each of the following parts of your body, take one or several breaths. Can you feel your breath in the front of your ribcage? In the back? On the sides? Can you feel your breath all the way up to your very top rib underneath your collarbones? How do your collarbones, your arms, and your shoulder blades move with the breath? Can you feel your diaphragm? In which places?

4 Follow your breath further down from the ribcage to your belly, your sides, and your lower back. Then follow it to your pelvic floor. What happens here when you breathe?

5 Notice how your bones feel. Then your feet, legs, and hip joints, your pelvis, your spine, your ribcage, arms, and head.

6 Roll back up slowly and observe: How are you feeling? How does your breath feel? How do you perceive yourself and your environment? What emotions are present?

7 If you like, you can now bring your torso down with a straight back. Just fold at your hips and let your torso drop down. What is different here? Can you hang lower like this? What's different now in your hip joints, the legs, the pelvis, the spine, the ribcage, the arms, and the head?

8 Roll back up slowly and sensuously; then observe the effects on your body.

PRACTICE 46: Reality Check

Observe your pelvis during the course of a day. When do you tense it? In which places? In the pelvic floor? In one or both sacroiliac joints? In one or both hip joints? What can this teach you about yourself and the situation? Do you have time for one of our relaxation practices? Then do it. By now, your body knows what it needs.

Try to do a Reality Check for a whole day. Set a timer that goes off every hour. Each time it does, check in with what your pelvis is doing.

Tip

PRACTICE 47: Drop the Pelvic Floor

Now that you can perceive your entire pelvic floor, you can also relax it completely. Relaxing the pelvic floor not only feels great; it's also an essential self-regulation tool. It's a way to indirectly influence your autonomous nervous system, which, as you know, is otherwise outside of your conscious control.

> **Tip**
>
> Conscious pelvic floor relaxation is used in therapy and in leadership training to get into a state of "non-anxious presence" for situations with a lot of tension in which it's important to be conscious, calm, and centered.[55]

1 Perceive your pelvic floor in its entirety and deliberately relax it. In your imagination, let it sink down further and further toward the earth. Observe where you hold tension and let go more and more.

2 Sense into your body and notice how your belly relaxes as well, how your breath becomes freer, and how your face relaxes too. How are you feeling?

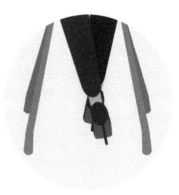

★ Relax your pelvic floor while you're having coffee with a friend, in a meeting with colleagues, or when you're having breakfast with your lover. Observe the effect it has on everyone present.

★ If you like, you can ask the people you're with whether they notice anything about you. I always hear that my presence has increased and that the person with me feels more comfortable. This technique works for women and men, and the more of us who know it, the more relaxed and deeper all of our relationships can be. Try it out when you're flirting, if you're stressed, in difficult conversations, in every life situation, and of course, during sex. This practice should be a staple in your Pussy Yoga toolkit.

Once you're used to it, you'll notice how much openness and supreme self-confidence this practice provides.

Tip

Pussy Practices

Now that you know your pelvic floor as the support structure in your body, we will also explore it through the pussy. Then we can do a few exercises purely for the pussy.

PRACTICE 48: Inner Retrospective—Feel the Practices in Your Pussy

It's time to experience everything you have learned from the inside of your pussy. Try the practices in this book with one finger inside your pussy. It won't work for every practice, but you'll get the idea.

1 You will need some peace and quiet, clean hands with your nails cut short (if possible), and some tasty oil from the kitchen. It's important to only put things in your pussy that you would also put in your mouth.

2 It's easiest to do this while sitting on a sofa, on an easy chair, or in bed. From there, you will be able to get into all sorts of positions.

3 Sit up and place an oiled finger as deeply inside your pussy as is comfortable for you. Relax and start by feeling what it's like in there.

4 Then go through all of practices in the book that are possible for you, and feel what happens inside your pussy. Feel with your pussy and feel with your finger. Do the practices for a few minutes.

5 Then relax fully, and notice how your pussy, your pelvic floor, and your finger feel.

6 Pull your finger out carefully and sense inside your pussy. Observe how your body feels now and how you feel in general.

If you're an experienced Pussy Yogini, your finger will be thoroughly kneaded after just a few minutes.

PRACTICE 49: Bring the Pussy Walls Together

1 While squatting, standing, sitting, or lying down, visualize where your vagina is located in your body, and breathe into it for a few breaths. Now imagine that you bring the right and left walls of the vagina together. Do it lightly, and pulse at first; then do it as firmly as you can. Practice this exercise with awareness and without using your sphincter muscles or focusing on the sit bones.

2 Observe which parts of your pelvic floor become active here and how far this little exercise can radiate into your body. Do you also feel a resonance through your entire body—in your heart, throat, or face?

3 Now consciously let go and observe how the tension slowly releases. To let go completely, breathe long, cool breaths into your pussy.

4 Next, begin pulsing with both sides or fluttering them as if you were applauding with them. Imagine a butterfly as you do so. Feel how this practice promotes circulation in your vagina as you begin to feel more and more. Relax completely.

5 Finally, bring together the front and back walls of your vagina. Observe how your entire levator ani integrates and aligns your pelvis. Keep your sphincter muscles relaxed at all times. Pay attention to resonance throughout your entire body: Where can you feel connections? In your mouth, jaw, and throat?

6 Let go and observe how everything gradually relaxes. This relaxation is especially important here. Your pussy can only be healthy and fully functional if she is completely relaxed.

PRACTICE 50: Pussy Elevator

This is a classic Taoist practice, which should only be used in moderation to avoid tensing up the pelvic floor.

According to the Tao, our pussy has reflex zones. Divided lengthwise and, starting at the bottom, these zones are (1) kidneys, (2) liver, (3) spleen and pancreas, and (4) lungs. The cervix at the very top of the vagina is connected with the heart. This explains why stimulating this area during sex causes many women to have very emotional orgasms.

1 Imagine your vagina is divided into these four zones from bottom to top; they lie on top of each other like rings. Now squeeze the bottom ring as if you wanted to crush something inside your vagina. Squeeze more and more until you reach 50 percent of your maximum tension. Keep this tension up, and go to the second ring,

tensing it to 50 percent as well. Then move on to the third and the fourth rings until you're contracting them all together. Keep your breathing relaxed.

2 Then let them go again, starting from the top to the bottom. Keep letting go for a while until you are completely relaxed. Repeat this exercise at most three times.

3 If you can, do the practice a bit faster, like a pulsation, and observe the energy in your body. Then let go completely.

4 Now join in with the breath. Inhale as you contract and breathe out through your mouth as you release the tension in your vagina. Allow an uncontrolled "ahhhh" to sound. Relax for at least as long as you practiced.

5 Then focus mentally on the upper part of your vagina at the cervix. Contract it slightly and notice what you feel. Activating or pulsing in this place gives me and many other women a feeling of whole-ness, peace, and grounding. Sometimes it activates by itself when I'm in a strong community of women. I suppose this is because there is a center of power here due to its connection with the heart.

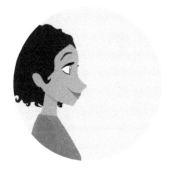

Back to the Roots

As you've read, our habit of sitting on chairs and sofas is one of the reasons that our pelvic floors are slack and lack mobility. But sitting has even more disadvantages for our overall health. Dr. James Levine, who has been studying the effects of sitting for over thirty years with his team at Mayo Clinic Arizona State University, argues that sitting is more dangerous to our health than smoking.[56]

Similarly, former NASA scientist Dr. Joan Vernikos compares the effect that hours of sitting every day has on our bodies with the drastic effects that weightlessness has on astronauts in space. Because muscles, bones, joints, and tissue do not support themselves against gravity in a seated position, they lose their strength and natural performance. Sitting also causes our gluteal muscles to do absolutely nothing, so eventually, they no longer fire when they're needed. This not only looks unattractive, but it also prevents natural pelvic alignment and pelvic floor tension, disrupting all of our natural movement patterns, such as standing, walking, running, and jumping.

While sitting, the muscles of our lower back have to hold the upper body upright without support from the strong gluteal muscles, which overloads and shortens them. At the same time, the abdominal muscles don't work effectively in the muscle network, so they become flabby and weak. The hips become immobile. The hip flexors shorten, and this forces the lumbar spine into a hollow back when we do stand. The upper part of the back sinks forward, the chest collapses, and there is a higher risk of herniated discs. In short, our bones need to bear weight to stay strong. Idle sitting leads to porous bones, especially in the pelvis and legs—and these are only the effects on our musculoskeletal system.

Too much sitting is also associated with type 2 diabetes, heart disease, fat metabolism problems, depression, and various types of cancer.[57] The studies on this topic are shocking.

Pregnant women are particularly affected, as their atrophied pelvic floor muscles are stretched up to a factor of four during pregnancy and childbirth. For a natural birth, the pelvis must be mobile. The coccyx must be able to nod to let the baby's head into the lesser pelvis first and then push it out with the opposite nod on the other side. It should also be able to move backward overall, which is rarely the case for women in the western world. This leads to episiotomies, cesarean sections, and a myriad of other pelvic floor problems after birth. Women who live in countries where squatting is common do not have problems to this extent.[58]

But it doesn't have to be like this! With Pussy Yoga, you have the tools to make sitting in the office more active, simply by using your pelvic floor. Another option is to change your position regularly while sitting. Try crossed legs, one leg placed on the seat, one leg with the ankle on the knee of the other, one leg folded under the buttocks, etc. It's important to keep getting up regularly as well: take a walk, hop, or dance. Taking short breaks in the office also helps restore your energy reserves.

However, the real solution is to minimize all of the sitting in our daily lives and return to our natural resting positions. We instinctively used them as small children before we were encouraged to sit on our little chairs. I see these resting positions often in Asia and Africa. People simply squat down, no matter if they're waiting, working in the fields, or selling something by the side of the road. When they later stand up and walk, they have a beautiful proud posture, no matter their age.

In our Essence of Bellydance courses, we have been using the deep squat since 2006 to stretch and activate the pelvic floor as well as all of the muscles, ligaments, joints, and fascia of the pelvis, legs, and back. I am happy to see that the deep squat is slowly becoming a trend among movement experts around the world. I would like to encourage you to integrate it as a vital part of your workout and into your everyday life. Please see the box "Squat for Number Two" for tips and ideas about how to do that.

Squat for Number Two

Now comes the inevitable second step for the brave. It's a bit adventurous, and even for me this information was rather annoying at first, but today I am super happy about this discovery. It's important for a healthy and fit pelvic floor, and it has far-reaching consequences for our overall health. Squatting for a bowel movement is healthier than sitting on the toilet. Research and studies have shown that many problems of our modern life arose with the spread of sitting toilets in the nineteenth century and are much less prevalent in cultures that still use squat toilets.[59]

There are many reasons for squatting down over the toilet. It's easier to empty the bowels and to do so more completely, thus preventing bowel cancer, inflammation of the bowels, and appendicitis. Squatting also protects the nerves that control the bladder and uterus from overstretching, and it seals the valve between the small and large intestine, preventing contamination of the small intestine. It relaxes the puborectal muscle as well, instead of allowing it to naturally close the anus while sitting. This muscle can make emptying the bowel in a sitting position so difficult that many people tend to squeeze. In the long run, pushing not only wears out the pelvic floor, but it's also the biggest cause of hemorrhoids.

PRACTICE 51: Deep Squat

1 Place your legs shoulder-width apart. Your feet can point out for now. Later on you can adjust and vary the position of your feet as you like. Next, slowly bend your knees and let your butt sink gently to the floor until it won't go any further without lifting your heels. If this is comfortable for you, skip to step 4.

Studies have shown that hemorrhoids can be reduced by taking up the habit of emptying in the squatting position. In pregnant women, squatting on the toilet prevents pressure on the uterus, and it also helps prepare them for a natural birth.

But since we largely don't use squatting toilets anymore, how can we solve the problem in an elegant way? There are various products that can be placed around or on the toilet to get into the proper squatting position, but as a minimalist, I have discovered the following method for myself: I put my feet directly on the toilet seat. This takes a little bit of practice in the beginning

and is probably easier for experienced Pussy Yoginis than for others. Experiment for yourself. First try a few dry runs so you'll be ready before it gets serious. The better you master the practices in this book and the deep squat itself, the easier it will be for you to climb onto the toilet. With this skill, you'll be able to squat on the toilet while you're at work or traveling as well.

Urinating of course is also healthiest in a deep squat, but you can still do it sitting down. It's important that you always pay attention to emptying your bladder completely in a single release and do not press at all. Just let go.

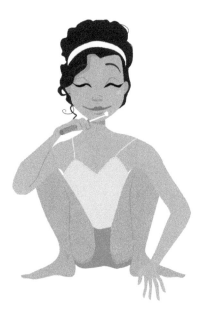

2 If a relaxed, deep squat is uncomfortable or impossible for you, try this trick: place a folded blanket or some books under your heels so you feel like you're wearing a pair of high-heeled shoes. Then let your butt sink down.

3 If this is still not comfortable or possible for you, stand in front of a door frame or any other upright structure that you can hold onto while moving very slowly into a squat (with or without a blanket under your heels). Do this exercise every day and gradually go lower. If it's hard, please don't give up. Mastering the deep squat and using it in your daily life is an important element of health for humans, and women in particular. Be patient with yourself, and know that all of the other practices in this book, especially the Pussy Yin series, will help you to become suppler in all the muscles and fascia that are involved here.

You can incorporate five minutes of deep squatting into your personal workout, and it's even better if you integrate it into your life in general. Get into the habit of squatting to read, work, and relax. Squat whenever you need a rest (instead of sitting on a chair), when you're watching films, when you're brushing your teeth, when you're using your smartphone or laptop, and especially when you're picking something up from the floor (instead of bending your back). Depending on how flexible you are, you could also squat on an office chair for a change of scenery, and you can even try it out as a position for your pelvic floor meditation.

Tip

4   Once you've reached one of the end positions mentioned in the previous three steps, relax here as long as it's comfortable. In particular, relax your pelvic floor more and more. Feel deep into your pelvis, your hip joints, your pelvic joints, and your spine, and notice how everything gradually releases. Breathe deeply and let go even more. Relax your spine.

5   If you feel pain, strain, or tension anywhere, come back up carefully. Walk around for a bit, and then try again. Pain is there to show you that your body is not yet capable of getting into this position easily, and you should never ignore it. If you have existing problems with your knees or your veins, ask your doctor for advice.

6 Experiment with different positions for your spine and arms.

7 If you can already squat comfortably, move your pelvis in all directions as you learned from the practices in this book. Stretch out your feet and legs as well, always with a sensuous and curious intention.

8 When you're done, stand up, leading with the head and keeping your spine straight. Use the strength of your butt and legs. Both squatting itself and getting into and out of squats trains your leg and butt muscles effectively and naturally, so it's good to do these often.

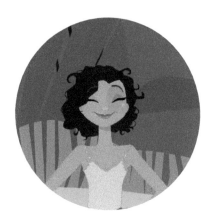

Pussy Yin

Pussy Yin practices are inspired by biomechanist Katy Bowman and the principles of Yin Yoga. They focus on restoring the natural balance of the pelvis and pelvic floor, and they also increase your mobility during sex.

Yin Yoga requires no warming up, so don't do it right after a strenuous workout. Instead it's perfect on its own or after your other Pussy Yoga practices. Hold these deep stretches for three to seven minutes. You can start with shorter periods to get used to the positions. Simply count seven very slow and deep breaths, which should give you an interval of about ninety seconds. If you increase your count to fourteen, you've reached about three minutes. Consciously relax all of your muscles and make the poses as comfortable and pleasurable as you can. Breathe into your muscles and fascia where you feel the stretch, and let go more and more. It should feel very good and restorative. You will notice that this letting go can put you into a deeply meditative state.

The long stretches in Yin Yoga release tensions and adhesions in the deep fascia, providing an effective, lasting stretch for our muscles, ligaments, and tendons. This will allow you to experience a new sense of mobility and natural alignment.[60] You can do our short Yin Yoga series any time to relax. It works amazing at night, promoting a restful deep sleep.

In between the practices, you can

★ lie down and observe (especially when you're stretching to relax before bed).

★ stand up and see if you notice an effect on your posture.

★ walk around gently to observe a difference in your movement flow.

★ go into a deep squat to see if this is now easier and more relaxed or if you can bring your feet closer together with your toes pointing more forward.

PRACTICE 52: Calf Stretch

Most women's calves have been shortened so much that it's almost impossible for them to walk in a way that suits their pelvis.

1 From a standing position, roll up a towel or a soft yoga mat, and place the ball of one of your feet on the highest point of the roll. Now slowly bring your heel down to the floor until you feel a stretch.

2 Straighten both knees. Keep the toes of both feet pointing forward with the legs hip-width apart and stand up tall in your usual walking position. Where did you place your second leg? For most of us, at first, it will be either behind or next to the leg we're stretching. The goal is to eventually bring your second leg to the front so its heel is the length of a step ahead of the toes of your stretching leg. Your posture should be relaxed and upright, not bending forward. Enjoy this deep stretch.

PRACTICE 53: Hamstring Stretch

1 Use your roll again and add a chair to lean on. Stand in front of your chair and bend your torso from the hip joints until your hands rest easily on the seat. This is like the Pussy Cow (Practice 12) but with straight legs. Now let your belly hang toward the ground. Your sit bones point toward the ceiling, and your pelvic floor is stretched open. You can hold your neck as an extension of your spine, or you can let it hang down. Can you feel the stretch in your hamstrings? If so, stay here, and keep stretching.

2 If not, use your rolled-up towel or mat as you did for the calf
stretch, and place it under the balls of your feet like before. Relax
and breathe slowly. Let go more and more.

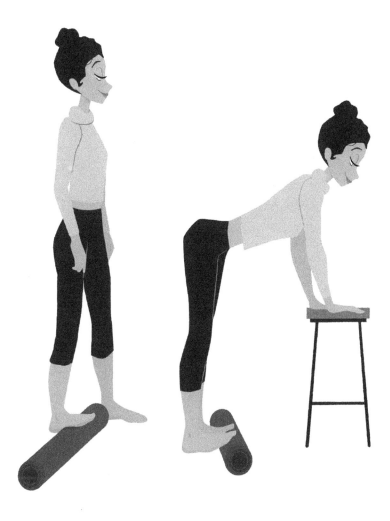

PRACTICE 54: Hip Flexor Stretch

1　Stand with the toes of both feet pointing forward. Slide one foot backward, bending the front knee and keeping the back knee straight. The heel of the back leg lifts off the floor: your pelvis and torso are upright and pointing forward. You will feel a nice stretch in your hip flexor.

2　If you don't feel enough of a stretch, keep going down further, but make sure your pelvis stays aligned and your sit bones sink downward. If you like, you could luxuriate in moving back and forth here to get the most out of the stretch.

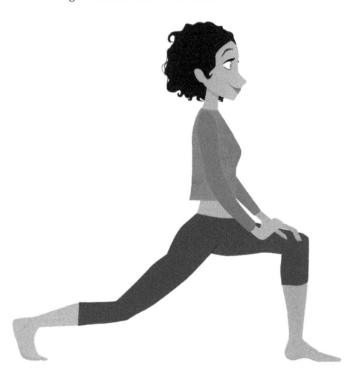

Exercises and Movement Patterns You Should Avoid

★ Studies have shown that sit-ups damage the pelvic floor because they push all of the organs against the pelvic floor with a lot of pressure.[79] Instead, try some whole-body movements, which strengthen abdominal muscles by integrating them. An example of a good exercise is the plank, along with its many variants. To do this, support yourself on your hands or lower arms and your toes while holding the rest of your body straight like a plank. Other good exercises are any in which you hang from a bar or a doorframe and pull your legs up using your abdominals.

★ Folding yourself like a jackknife from a lying position not only strains the pelvic floor and your spine in an unhealthy way, but it can also cause your abdominal muscles to tear along the middle at a place called the "linea alba." When you come up from the ground, it's better to spiral elegantly to the side while elongating your spine.

★ Avoid bending down with a rounded back to pick things up from the ground or do something near the floor because it puts strain on your spine. It's better to squat.

★ Try to not tuck in your belly. Many women do so unconsciously, but your belly doesn't just vanish when you contract it. Instead, it's pushed into your body, both upward and downward. This squeezes your organs, reducing their ability to work well. It also strains your diaphragm, which can then no longer allow a full breath, and it stresses your pelvic floor, which becomes slack or chronically tense. To be fully functional, the organs inside your torso should be gently stacked on top of each other and able to move freely. Instead of restricting your breathing, digestion, and all of your wonderful body's other biological and motor functions by sucking in your belly, there is a better way to look great. Do a few Essence of Bellydance upper body exercises every day to lift up your torso and stretch your silhouette with the power of your otherwise underused thoracic muscles. This also gives your organs a great massage, raises your energy levels, and makes you feel incredibly sexy and confident in your body.

PRACTICE 55: Lower Legs on the Wall

1 Find a free spot on a wall and lie with your legs pointing up against it. Now open your legs and let them slide down the wall gently to each side. Try to relax in this pose for up to twenty minutes by breathing deeply and calmly.

2 Optimize your position by tilting your pelvis so your tailbone moves toward the ground and you have a slightly hollow back. Observe how this affects your stretch.

3 Then turn your legs out, moving your little toes closer to the wall. Relax your pelvis and your pelvic floor.

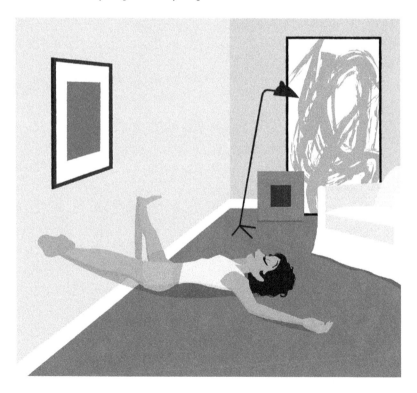

PRACTICE 56: Torso Stretch

Often, our pelvis tilts forward (anterior tilt) and creates a sway back to compensate for a rounded upper back. This is a great exercise for mobilizing your upper spine and your ribcage. It will also lift your chest and free your breath.

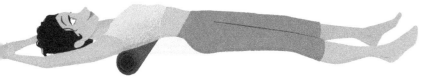

1 Have your rolled-up towel or mat ready. Then lie down across it at ninety degrees, with the roll placed just at the lower edge of your ribs. Relax here for a few long breaths.

2 Move down an inch or two so the roll now sits a little closer to your head and relax once more. Keep repeating and slowly rolling up as far as is comfortable. If necessary, you can support your head with your hands or a cushion.

3 If you have time and feel like it, you can roll back down. At the end, move off the roll and take some time to lie on the floor to observe the effects on your body.

If you want to mobilize your upper body even more, as well as aligning and strengthening it, I recommend the upper body exercises from EssenceBellydance.com or SensuousWorkout.com.
Complete your Yin Yoga session with a long, deep squat and lying down relaxation.

Tip

Discover the Anatomy of the Pussy

For a long time, the only known part of the clitoris was the clitoral glans at the upper end of the inner labia. But that's only the tip of the iceberg. Now we know that the clitoris consists of an entire system of nerves and erectile tissue: the little clitoral glans, two erectile structures that nestle into the front wall of the vagina, and two "legs," each 2.5 to 3.5 inches long, that reach far inside our body.

As an organ, the clitoris has only one function: to give us pleasure and orgasms. To do that, it has approximately eight thousand sensory nerve endings that are especially sensitive to touch and vibration.

However, the clitoris is not our only pleasure center. Our entire pelvis has nerves running through it, and every woman is slightly different in this respect. The pelvic nerve branches through every woman's pelvis in a different way, which is why some women are more sensitive on the tip of their clitoris while others are more sensitive in various places in their pussies or around their anus. As such, some women orgasm quickly from vaginal intercourse, while others need additional clitoral stimulation or prefer other kinds of stimulation altogether. Only 60 percent of women experience orgasms from intercourse, and oral sex is the easiest way to make a woman come. Every woman is different; there is no biological standard.

This delicate network of nerves is spread throughout the entire pelvis and is not confined to the superficial areas you can touch. How you experience your arousal and your orgasm is very personal to you and is determined to a large extent by your individual anatomy. In men, the

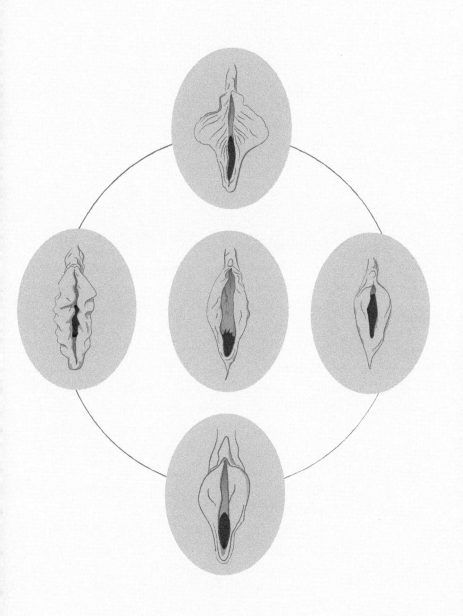

nerve structure, as far as we know today, is rather uniform. That's why they're often surprised that whatever worked well for their first girlfriend has no effect on other women. This can sometimes make women wonder if there's something wrong with them when they don't respond to their partner's caresses. But anything that's exciting for one woman could easily be boring, annoying, or even painful for another. It's your job to find out where your erogenous zones are and how you like to be stimulated. Only then can you show or tell your partner what you like in a sexy way.

PRACTICE 57: Waking Up Your Pussy

Have you ever looked at your pussy with a hand mirror or sat in front of a big mirror and looked at her from all sides? If not, now's the time! Wash your hands and prepare a tasty oil from the kitchen.

1 Make yourself comfortable with your hand mirror on a bed or a sofa, and begin exploring what your pussy looks like. Touch her, move her, and study her like a scientist. Take a look at the image of different pussies, and see whether yours appears there too. As you can see, pussies come in all sizes, shapes, and colors. There is no standard.

2 Take fifteen minutes to explore your pussy and her surroundings sensually with your fingers. Which areas are sensitive? Which are numb? Are there any tense places? What kind of touch does she like? What emotions come up? This is not about making any judgments or bringing yourself to orgasm, but rather it's an invitation to explore your pussy with curiosity. Get to know and love her in detail.

3   Next, we will dedicate fifteen minutes to the tip of the clitoris alone. With some oil on your finger, stroke your pussy from your vagina to the upper left side of your clitoris. As an experiment, caress this one area from top to bottom and side to side, over and over again. Make it a meditation and relax into it. Let your breath flow and observe what happens. This experiment is inspired by orgasmic meditation and could potentially tell you a lot about yourself and your relationship with joy, pleasure, and sex.

4   Next, we will venture inside. Slide your finger very carefully and slowly into your pussy. Explore what you feel and what emotions arise. How does the space inside your pussy feel? Wet? Warm? What shape does it have? Can you identify your urethra at the front? Can you reach the cervix? How does it feel? What does it feel like? Can you feel the area of the G-spot on the upper side of your pussy? Lightly press both the sides and the back. Try out other positions as well. See how your pussy feels in each position.

5   Let go and listen to your body. Observe whether anything has changed in you and in your pussy.

According to the teachings of the Tao, the pussy and the cervix have reflex zones that correspond to our organs and their associated emotions. It's also scientifically proven that your pussy, like the rest of your body, stores memories and trauma.[61] It's therefore possible that doing a pussy massage could bring up emotions. It may also change something in you, liberating you in a way you can't explain. Go with it, and trust in the healing power of your own body and intuition.

You can also trust in the natural healing abilities of your partner. They don't even need to know. Simply trust that everything your pussy experiences in a state of love, intimacy, and joy heals her.

PRACTICE 58: Pussy Meditation

This meditation is best done lying down, maybe as a ritual for waking up or falling asleep and anytime you like in between. Place one hand on your pussy and observe how she's feeling. Warm? Cold? Pulsing? What's her mood?

You can do this intimate meditation at any time and in any place. Notice your pussy in every possible situation and feel how she moves with your breath. Notice how soft and tender she is.

Expert help

If you still have difficulty finding your pelvic floor after dedicated practice, you may need individual support where you can, for example, practice with an intravaginal probe and a small monitor.

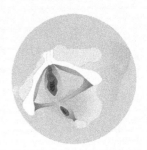

Sensuality
and Sex

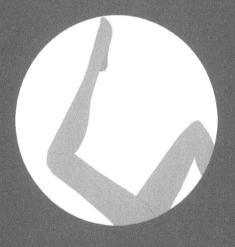

Really Good Sex

Like many other women, I've had consciousness-expanding experiences during sex. We suddenly feel flushed with love, one with everything, we're more present and clear, and we are filled with joy, inspiration, and lust for life. But is that the case for all women, and are there any scientific explanations for it?

Why Are Good Sex and Orgasms So Important for Us Women?

During the female orgasm, the regions of the brain that are responsible for self-perception, inhibitions, and self-regulation are temporarily deactivated.[62] This can mean that women feel incredible euphoria, love, and connection, not just in relation to their partner but also to themselves and to all of life. States of mind that are usually connected with spiritual experiences—a deep sense of peace, life-changing insights, creative breakthroughs—can arise from our orgasmic experiences. Sex can therefore be practiced as a spiritual path. Maybe you've had spiritual experiences during sex or other moments in your life. If so, you can look forward to more of them through Pussy Yoga; if not, there may be some empowering surprises in store for you.

In her investigation of the work and lives of female writers, artists, and philosophers from 1850 to 1930, Naomi Wolf found that there is a direct connection between each woman's sexual awakening and her creative breakthrough. Feminist artists and revolutionary thought leaders like Anaïs Nin, Georgia O'Keeffe, Hannah Arendt, Charlotte Brontë, George Sand, and Gertrude Stein were creatively, sexually, and intellectually freer than their contemporaries at a time when women had few rights.

Their sensual awakening was often accompanied by a willingness to take risks in social and artistic fields. Once those women stepped into their power, there was no going back.

A neurotransmitter called "dopamine" is partly responsible for this cultural phenomenon. It regulates the blood flow to our internal organs and ensures that our erectile tissue and inner labia swell when we're aroused. During orgasm, dopamine is released in large quantities and activates our brain's reward center, which puts us into a euphoric state of intoxication. These processes in our brain have the same effect as taking cocaine. That's also why, at some point, we behave like addicts during sex: we can't stop until we hit the big dopamine release during orgasm, after which we can calm down again.

We love this dopamine kick. It stimulates us; it provides clarity, ambition, motivation, and energy for achieving our goals. Dopamine helps us make the right decision at the right time, and it makes us self-confident and determined. Because it reconnects us women to our power, Naomi Wolf calls it "the ultimate feminist chemical."[63] A woman with a high level of dopamine knows what she wants and cannot be manipulated or controlled.

When women are aroused by sex but do not reach orgasm, they become sexually frustrated, and the dopamine curve flattens out. If no discharge follows the build-up too many times in a row, a woman can lose access to her arousal. She'll become unhappy and irritated, especially in relation to her sexual partner. She'll lose her ability to take pleasure in sex, and her ability to take pleasure in anything. This is often accompanied by addictive behaviors and depression. But the good news is that you can get your dopamine kick without a partner too! You don't even need to have sex. Exercise, shopping, dancing, playing with kids and animals, laughing with friends, and good parties can all help to maintain your dopamine levels.[64]

Testosterone is released during sex as well. This hormone not only increases our excitement; it also gives us a direct energy boost and the courage to be more daring.

Serotonin is a neurotransmitter that gives us a feeling of satisfaction and contentment. It's the counterpart to dopamine, and it makes us feel blissful, cozy, and serene after orgasm. An increased serotonin level lowers our drive, our urge to move, and our aggression. It also dampens our emotions and paralyzes our sexual desire. Once our serotonin levels return to normal after sex, our brains release dopamine once more, making us sociable, active, and hungry for adventure and sex again.

Noradrenaline is the hormone responsible for the intoxicating state we feel when we fall in love. It lifts our spirits, increases our attention, dispels hunger and fatigue, and dampens pain.

Endorphins, the body's very own opioids, promote relaxation and our ability to let go during sex. The more we trust our partner and the more we feel desired, the easier it is for us to relinquish control to our body and become orgasmic. What's interesting is that endorphins are released in larger quantities during sex with familiar partners than during one-night stands.

The release of our body's own opioids leads to states that meditators refer to as "bliss" or "oneness with everything." These states are also described by people who've had near-death and out-of-body experiences (both of which are linked to the release of dopamine and opioids).

Isn't this wonderful? Whether alone or with a partner, sexuality is our own means to free ourselves—to feel alive, creative, and full of energy! It can unleash our self-confidence and our connection to our intuition, not to mention our access to spiritual experiences. All of this is naturally inherent in our bodies.

Sensuality and sex are not something we should put off for when we have more time. Sex can give us more power now—for everything we want to do.

Orgasms help us feel more connected with our partner, thanks to the bonding hormone oxytocin. Oxytocin is released during sex, as well as during cuddling and skin-to-skin contact. Oxytocin is also a natural painkiller and helps release stress. Plus, it ensures a good night's sleep and thus better regeneration.

While bad sex can plunge us into depression, good sex can make us dependent on our partner. Studies have shown that women react differently to good sex than men do. Among other things, women produce more oxytocin, and deep heart-opening orgasms can make us emotionally dependent on our partner. That's why women must choose wisely when they let someone near their pussy. We should not feel ashamed about falling in love with our sexual partners or only wanting sex with love. It's not naïve; it's a sign of self-respect. Women tend to take sex and intimacy more seriously than men, and it's not weak—it's our biology. But this doesn't mean we're at its mercy. The more we understand our body and how to deal with strong emotions, the freer we can be.

Other Women

With my female friends, sometimes even with women I've only met once—and of course in my workshops and teacher training courses—I experience how healing and inspiring it is to share openly. The prerequisite for this is vulnerability. Without it, encounters between women can be superficial status games where everyone tries to put on a perfect show while hoping to catch a glimpse behind the other's perfectly crafted facade. Encounters like this leave everyone feeling dissatisfied. Whether they flatter our egos or not, they preclude a deep connection because we're afraid to show ourselves as we are.

How Much Sex Should I Have?

According to Dr. Nan Wise, most of our problems with sex revolve around a social standard we cannot meet, either because we don't want to have sex every day or because we don't experience orgasms the way they're portrayed in women's magazines, movies, or pornography. According to the American Association of Sexuality Educators, Counselors, and Therapists, the most frequent first question for sex therapists is: "Is it normal that…?" Why does everyone want to be normal? As long as you're happy with what you do, how, and how often you do it, it's all good.

Sex is still such a taboo subject, and when women don't talk about it as openly as they could, they think they're the only ones who are different and weird. Insecurities lead to shame—and it's precisely this shame and performance anxiety that make them feel inferior and move them further away from a passionate, exuberant love life. Pressure creates stress, and stress makes female pleasure and orgasms almost impossible.

The solution here is your Pussy Yoga: to connect intimately with your body, to feel what your pussy wants, to recognize what your intuition is telling you—to learn to feel what stimulates you, who you really are, and what you really want.

When you open up, you can experience close connections and real exchange. You don't have to dish up problems for authentic connection. Just be yourself and honestly communicate your opinions and feelings. A study at the University of California Los Angeles has shown that women who come together and share experiences release the love hormone oxytocin, which not only gives us a satisfying sense of community but also relaxes and helps us to better manage our personal stress.[65]

And if you feel you can, share your journey with a girlfriend—you can share a good laugh over it and inspire each other at the same time.

How the Female Orgasm Works

If you know what actually happens in your body during sex and if you learn what promotes and prevents amazing orgasms, you'll have the power to enjoy better sex so you can come more often and more intensely. It will help you avoid your personal turn-offs and killjoys, creating the perfect conditions for great sex.

We know today that the path to female orgasm is not a linear one, as early researchers assumed when they watched heterosexual couples having sex in their laboratories in the 1960s. It's more of a constant feedback loop that can unfold very differently each time and can reach several climaxes.[66]

The first step is the decision to want to have sex. It can arise spontaneously from a desire for sex or from another need, such as the desire to be close to your partner or simply to relax and feel good.

In the first case, arousal is already present; in the second, it comes about through physical contact or intention.

Most women need erotic stimulation and seduction before they can physically and mentally surrender to sex. It doesn't matter whether we do the seducing or are the ones being desired and seduced. We must feel sexy!

When we're sexually stimulated, sensations in our body send signals to the brain. In joyful expectation, the brain then sends more blood to our genital area, generating a feeling of arousal there. The increased circulation makes our pussy swell, especially the labia and the clitoris. Everything becomes more sensitive. Our pussy gets wet, our breasts enlarge, and our nipples harden. We breathe faster and our heart rate goes up.

All of this in turn sends back ever stronger signals to the brain, but only if you allow the arousal and don't interrupt it. In women, this initial arousal phase can last from a few minutes to a few hours.

The next phase is the sensual phase, in which we perceive erotic stimuli with all of our senses. We enjoy the good feelings and want more of them. Pussy Yoga teaches you to perceive your body's sensations more consciously and to indulge in them.

This trains your body to be more sensitive to touch and pleasure. If you're the kind of woman who tends to be in her head rather than in her body during sex, you'll begin to find it easier to surrender to your body and your lust for sex. If you focus more on your body and all of your senses, you'll notice more pleasure signals, feel stronger arousal, and achieve orgasm more easily.

In this sensual phase, the blood flow to the walls of the vagina increases, so blood collects there. This allows your vagina to lengthen and narrow at the front, so in the case of heterosexual case, it can adapt to any penis size. Once everything is plump and pulsating, you're ready to take in a penis and enjoy sex. Many women don't get properly aroused before intercourse, which dampens the fun for everyone involved. The full swelling of your pussy also makes sex more intense for your partner, so extending foreplay really pays off for all parties.

On average, women can come in less than four minutes on their own, but with a partner, they usually need about twenty minutes of whole-body stimulation and another twenty minutes of direct genital stimulation to reach orgasm.[67] The process is so fragile that even the smallest disturbances can prolong or kill it.

This is why it's important to take your time and to enjoy your path to orgasm, knowing your partner is also enjoying your increasing pleasure. There's no need to rush into anything because when you hurry, you block the necessary physiological processes for ecstatic sex, setting a course for a shallow exchange that leaves you empty.

For women, as you probably know from experience, the path to orgasm can easily break at any stage. There's no point of no return for us. These breaks can be our own inhibitions, fears, and expectations, or they can be external disturbances. To become more orgasmic, it's important to consciously perceive and enjoy your rising excitement, to surrender yourself completely to feeling and passion, and to let go of any distracting thoughts that come up.

As your arousal increases, you may need more intense touch, and you may even crave touch that would hurt you if you were less turned on. Toward the end of this phase, most women need constant rhythmic stimulation. The intensity shouldn't decrease if they want to reach orgasm now. Any small change in intensity or frequency can cause us to "lose" our orgasm.

But at this stage, you can also consciously choose to shift down a gear because the more often you delay your orgasm, building ever more desire, the more intense it can be in the end.

Orgasm requires absolute letting go. Feel the waves of ecstasy build up in your body and give in to it. During orgasm, our heartbeat, blood pressure, and breathing speed reach their peak. In addition, our pelvic and vaginal muscles contract with a decreasing intensity. It's an intoxicating state in which thirty different brain regions are active.

Some women can even "squirt" (i.e., ejaculate a clear fluid) because we women have an equivalent to the male prostate in our paraurethral gland. It's normal and healthy, but it's not a sign of a special peak, so it's okay if you don't squirt.

After an orgasm, you may crave more orgasms immediately, and these can easily build on each other. At other times, your desire may ebb away, leaving you feeling satisfied and relaxed. Genital swelling lasts about thirty minutes in women. Then the muscles relax, and all organs return to their original state.

How we experience our passion and orgasms is individual and different each time. My orgasms have changed and intensified a lot during my lifetime, and I still experience moments that amaze me: *Oh, so that's an orgasm*. Orgasms can bring us spiritual experiences, realizations, and deep insights. We can let go of old blocks and completely rediscover ourselves.

> Day after day, Pussy Yoga will make you more familiar with your body, your instincts, your pelvis, and your pussy, helping you to feel sensual, sexy, and irresistible. It will also make your pussy stronger, more agile, and more sensitive. It will stimulate the nerve endings in your pelvis so they can send more and stronger signals to the brain. This makes your arousal more intense and enables you to have stronger, fuller orgasms.

Let Go!

Studies have shown that women who manage to immerse themselves in their sensual sensations during sex, surrendering completely to feeling, find it easier to reach orgasm.[68]

As you focus more and more on feeling, you'll notice that, from a certain point in time, your sensations and feelings will carry you away. An experience of letting go and losing control is essential for fulfilled sexuality. On paper, that sounds quite enchanting, but loss of control is something many women fear. If, for example, we experienced being at the mercy of our parents or teachers when we were children, we can have a need for total control of our experience.[69]

To fully enjoy sex and become orgasmic, we must first let go of orgasm as a goal, focusing entirely on our feelings and enjoying the path without knowing the goal. Every time you trust in your body and its wisdom while making love, your brain strengthens those new neural pathways, so inevitably, you learn to move more and more toward a sensual orgasm. But the orgasm itself is always a gift. To experience it and feel fully satisfied, it can only be allowed, never forced.

See your sensual life as a practice and go deeper and deeper. How does it feel when your partner strokes your back? How does your partner's body feel on your skin? Surrender completely to the experience. Sense and savor every moment. And don't worry if images flash through your head or if you keep thinking of the office. As in meditation, notice the thoughts and then turn back to feeling. Getting annoyed about your thoughts only distracts you from the present moment.

Most likely, you'll reach an orgasm this way, but even if you don't, this practice pays off. Half an hour in this state of feeling and ever more feeling will bring you greater relaxation and more intimacy with your partner than if you got your partner off with your standard tricks, leaving nothing for yourself. Having relaxed into sensation, you'll feel like you've had a good massage or meditation session at the very least, and at best, you'll experience a mind-blowing orgasm. In any case, your partner will enjoy a sensual and sexy lover. In the orgasm-hunting scenario, you probably won't feel satisfied, and you'll blame yourself or your partner for "just not being good in bed." You may even question your relationship.

For a long time, I found surfing fascinating. *Gliding so freely over the waves must be an awesome experience*, I thought. But whenever I lived near a good surfing spot, the learning curve suddenly seemed too steep. I watched beginners as they constantly and awkwardly fell off their boards, and on top of that, you always had to paddle out while making sure you weren't being hit by the oncoming waves or rammed by other surfers. This seemed too bothersome to me.

But once my instinct to want to surf triumphed over my petty concerns, I tried it out, and I realized that once you get hooked, you just do whatever you have to do to catch the next wave. You paddle out, wait for a wave, jump on your board, and surf until the wave runs out or you fall off. Then you repeat the whole thing from the start, again and again, until you're completely exhausted and satisfied.

The elemental experience of nature and their body's abilities puts surfers in a state of nonthinking. A feeling of flow develops without any meditation technique. You just do it instinctively. And the same is possible with sex. Forget orgasm as a goal and simply do what brings you and your partner pleasure. Just do it! The more you learn to stay with your sensations, the more orgasms will come into your life.

Do What You Want

Claire Cavanah, the founder of feminist sex shop Babeland, coined the saying that "women learn to compromise before they learn to come." And herein lies a problem for all concerned: for sex to be hot, authentic, and true, you should touch your partner in a way that also turns you on. Stroke their body and notice how it feels. What are you in the mood for? What would you like to do with them?

If you only touch your partner the way you like, you'll find them sexier, which in turn will turn you on even more. Your partner will feel desired by you—and there's nothing more erotic than being desired by your partner and feeling this openly. For a man, a woman who wants him is far sexier than a woman who only tries to please him or succumbs to his touch, body, and energy. That doesn't mean, of course, that you shouldn't touch your partner exactly the way they like it, but it's about the intention. Try it sometime and feel the difference. Often, women are so accustomed to pleasing others that they cannot see the power they can unleash when they simply do what they love.

Safety, Relaxation, and Orgasms

We women need to feel secure and to trust in our partner before we can let go in bed and experience orgasms. And all humans need a sense of security in order to be creative and live their life with confidence and ease. This contradicts a persistent myth in our society, which says that security makes us lazy, losing all ambition, and that we have to push ourselves hard to be successful. It also says that too much security and love in childhood spoils children and makes them dependent on others. But the exact opposite has been proven to be true, time and again, by research since the 1970s.[70] Only once we calm our nervous system and our body feels safe can we relax and develop the capacity to have fulfilling relationships, to enjoy beauty, to learn, and to live creatively, be it in science, art, business, or spirituality. Feeling safe optimizes human behavior by eliminating the ancient defense mechanisms of our nervous system (fight, flight, freeze) and supporting social behaviors. It promotes mental and physical health.

Children who lack the feeling of security in their childhood often have behavioral and learning problems. They don't feel safe in the company of others and are afraid to allow too much emotional closeness or touch. They fear the exact elements that are needed to build trusting social relationships. When children grow up with a sense of security, love, and acceptance, however, they become more independent, courageous, and curious. They are more creative and embark on their own adventures without clinging to their parents and to what they know.

How can we act on these findings and strengthen our sense of security?

Find Your Own Femininity

In interviews, I'm often asked what femininity means to me. Most people find me very feminine. They see the work I do with women or rediscover their own femininity through my work, so they want to know my thoughts on the subject. They want to grasp it intellectually and integrate it into their world view, because femininity is a conflicting issue for most of us.

But I've always found categorization odd. I don't think it's helpful to the situation of women and anyone who is between the sexes in our society.

In fact, I resist this question. I think it holds us back from just being ourselves.

I don't find it productive for women to consciously move, dress, or behave in what is considered a more feminine way because they think this will get them closer to their essence as women. Instead, I encourage them to feel their pussies and their bodies, which are after all female animals, and to follow their instincts. Then they'll reach for a flowery dress or a pantsuit, depending on what feels authentic to them, and they'll do the things that are good for them, feel natural to them, and bring them closer to their personal essence and goals.

They choose to be flight attendants, politicians, or engineers according to their instincts and abilities. They'll be dominant in some situations but gentle and yielding in others. They'll cry or fight. They have a whole range of behaviors that are authentic to them, and they don't try to conform to a social construct that, no matter how old and widespread, is after all just a stereotype. When they draw from within, they do not reduce themselves to clichés of femininity. Instead, they express themselves as free human beings.

Feminism

When I was little, I wondered why women weren't allowed to become priests, why housekeeping always fell on our shoulders, and why we were the ones who took care of the children when a couple separated and the men were no longer in the picture. Later, I read Simone de Beauvoir and experimented with "collecting" men the way many men collect women. I fought not to be labeled a slut for doing so. It was a fight I couldn't win, but gradually, I learned to put my needs and goals above what others thought of me. I examined my own acquired beliefs about my role and my options as a woman, and I tried out many things.

I studied architecture, a traditionally male profession, and at the same time danced the most feminine of all dances, confidently using my sensuality to captivate audiences emotionally. I would call myself a feminist, but only in view of my conviction that women and men are equal human beings and should have the same rights in every respect. I cannot bear the victim role in which some feminists cast themselves and the rest of us women, accusing men of malice and exclusively dominance-oriented thinking.

Looking at human history, it's evident that every group, whether defined by gender, race, or social class, has always sought to defend its privileges from other less-privileged groups.[71] Therefore, it's important that we insist on equal rights for ourselves and for all women across the world. But I don't think that women are better people than men or that the world would be a better place if women were in charge. Which gender is better is a question that does not move us forward, but rather it divides us. In addition, it fuels an unconscious fear of trusting men, which can prevent us from completely opening up in our relationships and letting go during sex.

In 1994, the neurologist Dr. Stephen Porges published a groundbreaking discovery: we humans have a neural pathway that goes directly from the brain stem to the heart.[72] In the brain stem, this nerve is connected to the muscles of our face and head. The muscles we use to speak and hear, along with the expressiveness of the face and physical gestures, are thus connected to the nerve that directly regulates our heart. This feature gives us the opportunity to interact directly with our body and create a relaxed physical state that enables health, growth, and regeneration.

In order to lead a healthy life, our body needs something that Dr. Porges calls "cues of safety." We get those cues of safety from ourselves, but we also look for them constantly in our environment and especially in the people around us. In social situations, our body unconsciously scans our counterpart's energy, facial expressions, and posture for signs that indicate uncertainty or security for us. That is why we feel so comfortable with some people and find others exhausting or even disturbing. Porges calls what happens between two or more people "coregulation."

The better our body coregulates itself with other bodies, the better it's able to regulate itself over long periods of time. It becomes more resistant to signs of stress. This is how partners who feel safe, secure, and loved in their relationship have no problem being separated from each other for a while without having to exchange text messages all of the time. The more intimate, open, and good-natured we are with our friends, partners, and families, the more effective coregulation becomes. Intimacy is a state in which we can show ourselves fully without defenses and get the feeling that we're completely okay. Only then do we feel safe and accepted; only then can we also open up and fully let go during sex.

But what can we do if we're far from this state? Telling anxious and stressed people to just relax and let go is counterproductive. It implies that they are to blame for their condition, and it signals that they're not okay, which makes them tense up even more. If they could feel safe and relaxed, they would—because people naturally want to relax but often can't. What those insecure and anxious people really need are signs of security—signs that they're okay the way they are now and that everything is fine the way it is.

This is especially true for our relationship with ourselves and with our body.

Dr. Porges recommends self-love and self-nurturing. The first step you can take to feel safer and more relaxed is to meet your body with respect. If you're angry with your body because it reacts to stress naturally and contracts—or because it doesn't want to have sex or doesn't allow orgasms—you're sending it signs of rejection. This stresses your body and causes it to mistrust you, so you shut down even further.

Don't try to hide your nervousness. Feel it and own it. This not only breaks the vicious circle of mistrust in your body, but it will be perceived as more authentic, courageous, and sexy by others. In our society, we learn to control our body, but if you try to suppress your body's signs of stress, it will only feel more threatened and subliminally signal fear. We all notice when ease is just a pretense; our bodies sense when others are stressed. Oftentimes, we can't put our finger on it, but that person seems fake to us. We get a feeling that we cannot trust them. As a result, they become less attractive than they would be if they shared their state openly.

Another thing you can do is to interact more with people you trust. The effect is most immediate in live situations. Go meet friends in real life. Video calls, phone calls, or texts are, in descending order, a poor substitute. The most effective forms of coregulation are playing, cuddling, and sex. Unfortunately, these are the activities we don't deem important in our hectic lives, putting them off until later, when we have time. But these seemingly unproductive activities are not trivial, and they are not distractions. They're essential for our emotional health.

Allowing Emotions and Intensity

We all want to feel good and avoid bad feelings, but perceiving emotions is a holistic ability. You're either all in or all out. If we suppress fear, sadness, shame, and anger, we become emotionally numb and can also no longer fully feel love or joy. Without emotional intensity and open intimacy, our relationships and love life lose their depth and meaning. Our lives become flatter, duller, and maybe even depressing. Forced positive thinking is, as you know, no way out of the situation. It only worsens our nonacceptance and drives us deeper into a downward spiral.

We lose not only our vitality and joy for life but also access to our intuition, the internal system that tells us what we really want and what we don't want. Negative feelings are necessary; they're catalysts that show us what we don't like. They show us, for example, that we don't like to be treated in a certain way or that we don't trust a particular person or that we're not satisfied with the life decisions we've made so far. All of these are important insights on our way to a fulfilling life.

When we learn to handle unpleasant emotions by giving them space and letting them flow through us, we grow beyond ourselves. We update our self-image and remain emotionally open to passion and love. This gives us an emotional freedom that allows us to make the right, courageous decisions in our lives despite uncomfortable emotions such as fear, anger, or shame.

And what's the solution here once again? Where do emotions happen? Where do you feel loneliness, disappointment, or pride? Emotions take place in our body. We perceive them with the sense we call introspection. Pussy Yoga strengthens this sense together with the other senses that connect your body and your mind.

We could all use a few more techniques to help us get deeper into our inner world and, in turn, perceive our body better. If you get more intimate with your body, especially with your pelvis and pussy, you'll notice that your body also stores old emotions.[73] Everything you have ever experienced has also been experienced by your body, and the stronger the emotion that accompanied the experience, the clearer the memory. Memories of these experiences can arise like flashes of thought, visions, or emotions. Allow everything to happen, but don't hold on to it, and try not to analyze it. Your body has its own wisdom and healing power, which you can discover through Pussy Yoga.

The following will help you deal with emotions that can come up through your Pussy Yoga practice, and it will also help you work with unpleasant emotions that hold you back in life. Whenever we try to suppress our emotions, when we're afraid of feeling them, they actually start to run our lives. If we try to avoid feeling fear, for example, the avoidance can keep us from stepping out of our comfort zone, getting to know great people, making important life decisions, or opening up during sex. Meanwhile, daring to actually feel the fear, getting to know it and doing whatever we were fearing, would expand our comfort zone and give us the thrilling feeling of uncertainty, excitement, growth, and mastery.

PRACTICE: Emotional Freedom

Whether you have a strong emotion or just want to listen to yourself to become more emotionally alive, the following process from Russ Harris's book *The Happiness Trap* is a wonderful way to get in touch with yourself.[74]

This process may transform negative emotions, but it doesn't have to. Our goal is not to get rid of unwanted emotions but to learn to live an exciting, fulfilling life with *all* of our emotions.

1 Observe what you can feel in your body. Scan yourself from head to toe. Can you spot anything particular or maybe unpleasant? Now concentrate on what bothers you the most. For example, it could be a sluggish feeling in your chest. Observe it with curiosity, like a scientist. See where it begins and ends. Where exactly are the outlines of the sensation? What form does it take in your body? Does it have a pulse or a vibration? Is it light or heavy? Warm or cold?

2 Breathe into this sensation. Breathe deeply and slowly, and then exhale completely. Breathe as slowly as you can. Slow breathing helps reduce the tension in your body. It can be like an anchor in the storm that centers you.

3 Now open up to the feeling, and let it expand in your body. Give it more and more space.

4 Allow this feeling to be there. Welcome it, even if it isn't easy for you. Remember, we aren't trying to change our emotions. The goal is to make peace with them. Fighting emotions is a painful waste of energy. It's exhausting. Only acceptance brings you peace, and the feeling will have less power over you.

5 Once you're at peace with this emotion, you can look for more sensations until you feel satisfied. Or you could just relax and let it be.

Tip

I love to do this practice anytime and anywhere, especially if I get wrapped up in thoughts and lose connection to the moment. Try it while meditating, riding a bike, standing in line, walking in nature, or falling asleep in bed. Listen for any kind of emotion, and you'll either discover the root of a wound or let irrepressible joy or love expand in you.

Enjoying positive feelings also requires discipline. I used to catch myself repeatedly analyzing every trace of genuine joy to understand what the reason was and how I could capture that joy and make more of it at the push of a button in the future. But it's precisely this thinking that took me away from the feeling of joy. It brought me from an instinctive sensual existence into analytical problem-oriented thinking.

Usually, there wasn't any particular reason for feeling good. It was just a state of joy. Analyzing the circumstances of my life only showed me that I had a lot to do, so I started planning and optimizing again. Because these thoughts felt so much more real and useful than the baseless feeling of joy, I went along with them.

From my work with women, I know that many of us feel this way and that the inability to simply relish the expansive feeling of joy is one of the reasons we can't relax and just be happy. The next time you notice a positive feeling flowing through you, enjoy it. Let it expand and flow in the awareness that there will always be new moments like this one, and that the desire to hold on to such moments will nip them in the bud.

Enjoy your emotions and let them flow the next time you make love. Simply sweep away your thoughts. There will be time for them later if they're really that important. This trains you to live in a state of joy.

In Pussy Yoga, we approach ourselves with curiosity and love by asking how we're feeling physically and emotionally. Intellectual analyses and monologues are not helpful here. You've probably been in situations where you wanted to talk about a problem you're experiencing, but the other person thinks they know what you want to say and starts giving you unsolicited advice or blames and belittles you. You feel misunderstood and will certainly not open up to this person again. That's how your inner self feels if you don't respect it and really listen to it like a good friend.

When you learn to tune in and listen to your inner world, you'll get to know your true self, gain direct access to your intuition, and step into your true power. When you observe yourself and your emotions, don't jump into analysis. Really listen. Most of us are quite judgmental and not particularly friendly to ourselves. We talk to ourselves in a tone we would find offensive in others. This negative self-talk stresses our body, and it perceives this stress in the same way it perceives stress from life-threatening situations. Then we not only feel the initial uncomfortable feelings; we feel threatened on top of it. The way out is to step back from the merciless carousel of thoughts and judgments and turn toward feeling and relaxing. Once you're relaxed, you have access to all of your emotional, mental, and physical resources: your inner wisdom.

The Female Rhythm

For women, our sense of pleasure and our self-confidence change not only with the circumstances of our lives, but also with our cycle. On our fertile days, we feel invincible and sexy. We flirt more, we're more assertive and adventurous, we dress sexier, and we're perceived by men as more attractive. Women with a natural cycle (without hormonal contraception) have a clear advantage here.[75] In the time before and during our period, we feel more vulnerable, and some of us are really down. If we don't know our body and its natural rhythm, we can easily slip into negative thought spirals, and our self-confidence can drop below zero. But it doesn't have to be like this. If you're aware that your body goes through these cycles of hormonal fluctuations, you can relax and sail through them. You can rest assured that every phase will pass and enjoy the ride through the ups and downs without attaching too much meaning to them. Feeling mellow and vulnerable for a few days doesn't mean that you won't feel highly energized and invincible next week. You can do this intuitively and share experiences with your girlfriends. For example, I've noticed that I'm full of energy and self-confidence on my fertile days, but I'm also more superficial and impatient. I'm not as empathetic, open, and loving as I am when I'm bleeding. My period is my time for deep love and strong connections, for insights and visions. The time before my period is not my favorite part of my cycle, but eagerly anticipating every sign of my bleeding is a bit like the time before Christmas.

You'll be pleased to hear that Pussy Yoga will help balance your hormones, stabilize your cycle length, and reduce or eliminate PMS and cramps. It has also helped bring about many longed-for pregnancies.

Observe how your body and your hormones change over the course of your cycle. Apps like Lily or Hormonology make this easier. Keeping track of your cycle is a wonderful way of using your senses to understand and love your body and to realize it's magic.

However, I advise against obsessing and planning your whole life around your cycle, as has become popular in recent years. It makes you less free. You can master important negotiations and public speaking with the specific energy of every phase of your cycle. Knowing your cycle makes you more understanding of your body's resources and more compassionate with yourself.

If you don't have a natural cycle because you take hormones like the pill, I recommend you watch the interview I did with Dr. Dorothee Struck, in which we discuss everything you need to know. You can find this interview and other Pussy Yoga goodies at Coco-Berlin.com/en/pussyyoga.

Accepting the change into a new phase of life and personality is also the best approach for menopause. A new study by the Dresden University Hospital for Psychotherapy and Psychosomatics presented a menopausal symptom questionnaire to 1,400 women aged between 15 to 95. It found that typical symptoms of menopause also apply to many younger or older women. Apart from hot flashes and sweats, the other symptoms do not peak in menopause. Women do not become more irritable, discouraged, forgetful, or anxious when the estrogen level in their body drops. The study found that whether women sleep poorly or have less desire for sex depends rather on factors such as self-efficacy, education, income, partnership, and employment.[76]

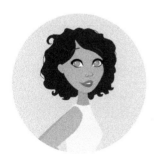

Open Senses, Open Heart

As Albert Einstein once said, "The most beautiful thing we can experience is the mysterious. It is the source of all true art and science. He to whom the emotion is a stranger, who can no longer pause to wonder and stand wrapped in awe, is as good as dead—his eyes are closed."[77] We can only feel this mystic feeling when we turn on our senses.

Meditation, dance, and yoga are all good tools, but it isn't actually what we do that matters; it's how we do it. If we pursue any of those disciplines with our eye on the prize and don't enjoy the path—the activity itself—we keep ourselves from the true experience of flow. If, on the other hand, we devote ourselves to these disciplines (or anything else in life) with open senses and a state of wonder, we'll experience states of flow and bliss.

You can practice any mundane activity in that way: making your bed, shopping, cooking, and of course, making love.

Sensuousness is always equated with sexuality, but I use the term as a fundamental attitude toward life. It's a state of being in which we consciously perceive ourselves and our environment with open senses in a state of wonder. In this state, we're deeply rooted in our instincts, our intuition, and our emotions. We truly live in our body and in the present moment, and we feel the vibrancy of life. It's a state of intensity, joy, and love.

Living in the Now

When we pay attention to our sensory perceptions, we are present. We perceive what is right now without thinking about the past or worrying about the future. That doesn't mean we run away from our problems; on the contrary, by allowing and facing all of the feelings that are present (as you learned in the Emotional Freedom practice) you won't need to run away from problems. By shifting your focus to the present moment and onto what is, you gain perspective without getting caught up in overthinking.

We can't solve everything intellectually, especially if our thoughts keep going in circles. Today, scientists believe that 90 percent of our 70,000 to 80,000 daily thoughts repeat themselves constantly and are not exactly helpful. Our body perceives fears about the future and memories of painful experiences from the past to be just as real as actual threats, creating unnecessary stress in the present.

The more often you dwell on threatening issues, the more stress you create in your body and the more you solidify negative patterns in your brain. For the most part, we're not even aware of our thoughts.

If you manage to step off the carousel of your thoughts every now and again or, better yet, for long periods of time, you'll learn not to identify too much with your thoughts. Consequently, you'll see more clearly and think more precisely.

When we learn to consciously switch our minds off, we also open ourselves to insights from our intuition, which, scientifically speaking, is our subconscious or implicit body knowledge. From a spiritual point of view, it's our soul and the higher consciousness that we're all part of.

In the Pussy Yoga practice section, we primarily train our potential for sensuous self-perception. Now I want to share some of my favorite sensuous tips for everyday life. They'll help you open all of your senses more fully and cultivate a strong sensuous attitude so you can savor every moment of your precious life.

There's no simple trick that leads to a sensuously satisfying life. The sensuous path is more of a lifestyle. The magic happens when you keep practicing it, but it's a true pleasure.

Your Sensuous Nature

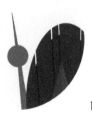

Nothing connects us to our senses, our body, and our instincts quicker than immersing ourselves in nature. Take your body, mind, and soul outside every day! Enjoy where you are and what you can sense, smell, hear, and see. Feel how your body is bare to the elements.

Whether you live out in the wilderness or in the urban jungle, let the weather seep into your soul. Dive in and feel the moisture of a fall evening, the sultry heat of summer, or the dryness of a cold winter's day. Soak up the colors of the ever-changing sky. Let the fresh breeze or the wild storm caress your skin and play with your hair. Listen to the leaves rustle in the trees or your steps on the gravel. Feel the energy of the nonstop traffic on the street.

Breathe in the fresh air deeply and take in the scents of nature. Smell the wind, the trees, the bakeries. Feel how you're part of everything. Take a walk without a destination in mind, and surrender to the wonder of nature, which surrounds you always, wherever you go.

Don't have time? Then switch on your sensuousness on the way to work or while you're shopping.

Fascinating Skin

Let's take a closer look at your skin. Examine it. What color is it? What kind of texture? Do you see veins? Hair? Wrinkles? Traces of your life up to this point? Isn't it fascinating?

Your skin is not just a 0.5- to 1.5-inch-thick beautiful shell that protects and holds your body together; it's also your largest and most versatile organ. On average, it has 18.6 square feet of surface area and weighs 22 to 30 pounds. Skin plays an important role in metabolism; it breathes, detoxifies, and perceives the environment. It adjusts to the climate inside and outside of your body. Through your skin, you communicate the state of your emotions and your health. Its millions of nerve endings not only enable you to feel tenderness or arousal, but also allow activities that require dexterity, like writing.

PRACTICE: Increase Skin Sensitivity

1 How are you aware of your skin? Where can you feel it now? Can you perceive your whole skin at once?

2 Feel the slight breeze on your neck with your skin. Feel where your clothes touch you. Feel the ground beneath your feet...

3 Now touch your left arm with your right hand. Notice the skin on your hand and also the skin that it touches. How does it feel? Isn't it great to live in your own skin?

Body Care Rituals

Do you rush into the shower in the morning and scrub yourself down until you're clean, or do you enjoy a private cleansing and caring ritual? A sensuous care ritual doesn't take more time because it's something you're doing anyway, so you may as well enjoy it. Use it to wake up every part of your body and connect with your sensuousness.

Once again, it isn't about what you do but how you do it. How would you like to be treated when you go to a luxurious spa? Treat yourself that way every day.

PRACTICE: Time for Yourself

1 Take your time feeling the refreshing water, whether you're quickly washing your hands or taking a shower. Imagine the water cleansing and refreshing you inside and out.

2 Massage your body as you shower. Enjoy every part of your body.

3 Dry your body off with care.

4 If you moisturize, massage your body and your feet attentively.

5 As you brush your teeth, notice how you clean each and every tooth with your toothbrush. Imagine massaging every tooth and your gums to become healthier and more beautiful.

6 If you wear makeup, apply the products with care, aware that you're enhancing your natural beauty.

All of this is something I have to remind myself of again and again because I was brought up to not be vain and to do everything quickly and efficiently. It isn't vain to treat your body with love. After all, the way we look at ourselves is how we look at others.

Massages

A good massage is like a reset for the senses. Do you believe massages are a luxury? A decadent pleasure for special moments?

Then imagine how you would feel if you received a massage every week. Yes, you would be more sensuous and relaxed, but according to scientific discoveries, you would also be healthier.[78] Massages are humanity's oldest healing method. Every culture has developed its own forms based on different theoretical principles. Try them all out, and if it's too expensive for you, take a massage course with your partner or a friend and then swap massages with them. Massage is a very personal art that human beings can share with one other.

Self-massages are a wonderful addition to your self-care rituals.

PRACTICE: Loving Whole-Body Detox Massage

1 With silk gloves before showering, brush your limbs with long strokes, circling at the joints and lymph nodes.

2 First, sweep out your face and neck from the midline toward the sides and in the direction of the heart. Then go up from the left foot to the pelvis. Repeat for the right leg and then your butt, all the way up to the heart.

3 Go in a circle around your belly, clockwise in the direction of your digestion.

4 Now stroke from the left fingertips to the shoulder, then the right arm, and the back of the neck. Sense with your hands how your body feels, and at the same time, enjoy the sensations of your own strokes.

You can do the exact same massage with your hands as you soap yourself in the shower or as you moisturize afterwards. Enjoy your body!

PRACTICE: Detox and Lifting for Your Breasts

A breast massage is a wonderful ritual for getting in touch with your sensuousness, learning to love your breasts, and keeping them lifted and healthy all lifelong. Breast massage helps your circulation in addition to stimulating lymphatic flow, which nourishes your breasts, detoxes your body, and reduces breast pain before your period. It even prevents cancer. Amazingly, this massage also stimulates the release of oxytocin. Remember our stress-reducing love hormone?

I do a mini breast massage for a few seconds or minutes several times a day, whenever I wake up, shower, or change my clothes. It's become a habit. I notice my breasts and take pleasure in their beauty, their health, and the lovely feeling I get from the massage.

Try the following techniques and follow your own flow. Trust your body. It shows you what it needs. Do each movement on both breasts before going on to the next technique. Repeat all movements for as long as you enjoy them.

1 Visualize the massage supplying your breasts with fresh energy while detoxing them at the same time. Enjoy their unique beauty and sensitivity.

2 Stroke them with both hands from the side, from underneath your arm to the nipple, again and again. Then stroke again from the point between your breasts to the nipples and then from below and from above.

3 Use your fingers or palms to go in circular motions over your
nipples.

4 Take your palms around the breast: move up on the inside, then
toward the sides and down, then back to the center and so on. Find
your perfect flow. Don't worry about pressing too hard. A firm massage will not stretch out your breasts, but instead, it will vitalize
and firm them. Next, circle in the other direction.

5 Draw small circles with your fingertips on the breast around the
nipple. Be curious about the tissues of your breast. This helps to
stimulate your lymphatic flow, which is your body's detoxification
system.

6 Move your right hand around both breasts in a figure-eight loop.
Change direction. Then use your left hand, again in both directions.

7 Place your hands around the lower edges of your breasts as if your
thumb and pointer finger form a bra's underwire, and stroke them
upward toward your nipples as if you were trying to squeeze something out of your nipples. You can imagine as you do this that you're
pushing old stagnant energy out of your breasts and shaking it off.

8 Hold your breasts the way you like best and feel into them. Enjoy
the sensations. Be grateful if you have two healthy and beautiful
breasts and that every massage makes them more beautiful, firm,
and healthy.

In Conclusion—Self-Acceptance

Pema Chödrön, a Buddhist nun and author, describes the wish for self-improvement as a subtle aggression against the being we actually are. We often believe that we're faulty in some way and must correct or at least hide our faults and quirks. But the opposite is true because our greatest weaknesses contain our greatest strengths. They are two sides of the same coin.

We do best if we courageously live out our strengths and keep an eye on our weaknesses so they don't lead us to destructive behaviors. It's important to know ourselves and to leverage what we have inside of us. For example, you might consider yourself to be reckless and inconsiderate, or you could embrace this quality and enjoy the fact that it enables you to take more risks and act bolder than others. It can be a strength that more conservative people secretly admire in you. At the same time, you make sure that you don't go overboard and thoughtlessly endanger yourself and others.

We can only step into our full power if we accept ourselves with everything that we are and courageously live what we are in our innermost being. Then we embody this wonderful human being that only we can be because we're all unique.

To live your potential and achieve your dreams, you must grow from strong roots. Don't try to contort yourself into the cookie-cutter shape of a perfect person. If you're dissatisfied with yourself right now, it's more likely that you're only twisted and bent down like a little plant that hasn't got the right care. If you turn back to yourself like a loving gardener and nurture and care for yourself, you'll come back to life and regain the energy to unfold your whole personality.

Authenticity is the one thing that makes us sexy and powerful. In search of it, we sometimes fall into the trap of limiting beliefs about ourselves that have been inculcated in us by our parents and society (such as, "I'm shy," "I can't come out of my shell," "I'm not charismatic," "I'm not athletic," etc.). Did you know that, for many years of my life, I believed I couldn't dance and had no sense of rhythm?

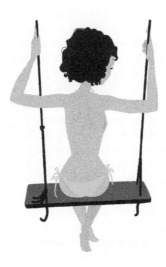

It started with a mocking comment by my father about my lack of rhythm. I immediately believed him and didn't dare to express my joy in music and dance in public for years.

But the passion I felt in my body when I listened to music was so great and, at the same time, so pure that I couldn't imagine there wasn't something to it after all. Secretly, I dreamed of dancing on stage and expressing the beautiful emotions I felt coming to life through the music.

In other words, my intuition set me on the right path. You already know how that story ended, and you hold my tools for self-discovery and empowerment in your hands.

I wish you a wonderful journey! Please let me know how it goes.

You can find me on social media.

YouTube: @cocoberlin
Facebook: @likeCOCO
Instagram: @cocoberlin_

If you use the hashtags #pussyyoga and #cocoberlin, I will find your posts.

Yours,

Coco

If you want to get in touch with me and other readers, or if you need more inspiration, you'll find everything you need in the bonus materials on Coco-Berlin.com/en/pussyyoga.

Acknowledgments

Thank you to all of my students, clients, and participants in my teacher training for your trust, your enthusiasm, and your feedback—and for sharing this work with others.

Thank you to all teachers, mentors, authors, and body workers for tirelessly researching and sharing your knowledge. Thanks to Dr. Dorothee Struck—your professional enthusiasm for my method and your review of the medical content in this book have encouraged me.

Thank you Rebecca Randak for recommending me to Komplett Media, my German publishing house. Thank you to Verena Schörner and Komplett Media for the complete artistic freedom and your trust in me. Thank you Heike Kmiotek for the illustrations. Thank you Lydia Kühn for the graphic design. Thank you Rebecca Darby for laying the foundation by translating my German book into English. My deep gratitude goes to Kat Pedersen and Anne Kavanagh for working with me tirelessly through the text again and again, giving Pussy Yoga so much love in editing and refining it until it finally sounded like me with better English. Thank you Lana Shlafer for bringing Anne into my life. Thank you Will Tyler for proofreading everything diligently and big thanks to Kat Pedersen for making sure every detail was perfect at the end. Thank you Heike Kmiotek for the illustrations and Lydia Kühn for the graphic design. Thank you Anton Khodakovsky for setting the layout beautifully. Thank you Kat Pedersen for encouraging me to publish Pussy Yoga internationally and directing the publishing and launch.

Thank you my soul mate and husband Christoph for your love and support. I am infinitely grateful for having met you eighteen years ago and our incredible journey through life together.

Thanks to the caring and responsible people in my family who did their best with what they had. Thanks to the bad and the ugly for ultimately making me a force for good.

Endnotes

1 Peter A. Levine, *Waking the Tiger: Healing Trauma—The Innate Capacity to Healing Overwhelming Experiences* (New York: Berkeley 1997). Bessel van der Kolk. *Verkörperter Schrecken: Traumaspuren in Gehirn, Geist und Körper und wie man sie heilen kann* (Lichtenau 2017).

2 Naomi Wolf, *Vagina: A New Biography* (London: Virago, 2012).

3 Moshé Feldenkrais. *Awareness through Movement: Health Exercises for Personal Growth* (Middlesex: Harper & Row, 1972, 1977).

4 Kaiser Permanente Division of Research, "One in Three Women Has Pelvic Floor Disorder," *ScienceDaily*, 5 (March 2008), www.sciencedaily.com/releases/2008/03/080302150723.htm. According to the Jean Lawrence study, 25 percent of women suffered from fecal incontinence, 15 percent from urinary incontinence, 13 percent had an overactive bladder, and 6 percent had sagging organs (that is, the uterus or the bladder slid down). According to the Neurological Urodynamics and Urology Institute, 29 percent of women will have more than one operation in their lifetime to correct pelvic floor problems.

5 David Wise and Rodney Anderson, *A Headache in the Pelvis: A New Understanding and Treatment for Chronic Pelvic Pain Syndromes* (San Francisco: Natl Center for Pelvic Pain, 2008). Robert M. Sapolsky, *Why Zebras Don't Get Ulcers*, revised edition (New York: St Martin's Press, 2004).

6 The word "vagina," in medical terms, only describes the canal between the vaginal opening and the uterus.

7 Eve Ensler, *The Vagina Monologues* (New York: Dramatist's Play Service, 2007). Regena Thomashauer, *Pussy: A Reclamation* (Carlsbad: Hay House, 2016).

8 Wikipedia, "Pussy," January 2018, en.wikipedia.org/wiki/Pussy.

9 Wikipedia, "Yoga," January 2018, de.wikipedia.org/wiki/Yoga.

10 Yuval Noah Harari, *Sapiens: A Brief History of Humankind* (London: Vintage, 2011).

11 Jonathan Isbit, "Health Benefits of the Natural Squatting Position," *Nature's Platform*, January 2018, www.naturesplatform.com/health_benefits.html.

12   Beate Carrière (Hrsg.), *Beckenboden, Physiothrapie und Training* (Stuttgart: Thieme, 2003).

13   John T. Cottingham, Stephen W. Porges, and Kent Richmond, "Shifts in Pelvic Inclination Angle and Parasympathetic Tone Produced by Rolfing Soft Tissue Manipulation," *Physical Therapy*, 68, no. 9 (September 1, 1988), 1364–1370, doi.org/10.1093/ptj/68.9.1364.

14   Jean M. Twenge, Ryne A. Sherman, and Brooke E. Wells, *Declines in Sexual Frequency among American Adults, 1989–2014 Arch Sex Behav* 46 (2017), 2389–2401, doi.org/10.1007/s10508-017-0953-1

15   Virginia Danielson, *The Voice of Egypt Umm Kulthum, Arabic Song and Egyptian Society in the Twentieth Century* (Chicago: University of Chicago Press, 1998).

16   C. Bibette, M. Roux, M. Lavergne, "Ägypten: Tugendwächter sind gegen Bauchtanz," ARTE GEIE, 2019, youtu.be/pJ2kCG1b4mY.

17   Frédéric Lagrange: Al-Tarab: Die Musik Ägyptens, Heidelberg: Palmyra, 2001. Joachim Bauer: Warum ich fühle, was Du fühlst: Intuitive Kommunikation und das Geheimnis der Spiegelneurone, München: Heyne Verlag, 2005.

18   Louise Barrett, *Beyond the Brain: How Body and Environment Shape Animal and Human Minds* (Princeton: Princeton University Press, 2011).

19   Barrett, *Beyond the Brain*. Almut-Barbara Renger, Christoph Wulf, Jan Ole Bangen, and Henriette Hanky, "Körperwissen, Transfer und Innovation," in Almut-Barbara Renger, Christoph Wulf (Hrsg.), *Körperwissen: Transfer und Innovation* (Berlin: De Gruyter, 2016).

20   Eric Franklin, *Beckenboden Power: Das dynamische Training für sie und ihn* (2002; repr., München: Kösel-Verlag, 2011).

21   Gerald Hüther, Wie Embodiment neurobiologisch erklärt werden kann, in Embodiment (Bern: Hogrefe AG, 2017).

22   Fatma Al-Maskari, "Lifestyle Diseases: An Economic Burden on the Health Services," *United Nations Chronicle*, December 2020, www.un.org/en/chronicle/article/lifestyle-diseases-economic-burden-health-services.

23   Hüther, Wie Embodiment neurobiologisch erklärt werden kann.

24   Moshé Feldenkrais, *Awareness through Movement*.

25 Bauer, *Warum ich fühle, was Du fühlst.*

26 Eugene T. Gendlin, in *Focusing* (New York: Rider, 1978).

27 Klaus Grawe, *Neuropsychotherapie* (Göttingen: Hogrefe, 2004).

28 Michael Eid and Randy J. Larsen, eds., *The Science of Subjective Well-Being* (New York: Guilford Publications, 2008).

29 G. E. Weisfeld and J. M. Beresford, "Erectness of Posture as an Indicator of Dominance or Success in Humans," *Motiv Emot*, 6 (1982), 113–131. doi.org/10.1007/BF00992459.

30 Maja Storch, Wie Embodiment in der Psychologie erforscht wurde, in *Embodiment* (Bern: Hogrefe AG, 2017).

31 Amy J. C. Cuddy, Caroline A. Wilmuth, and Dana R. Carney. "The Benefit of Power Posing Before a High-Stakes Social Evaluation," Harvard Business School Working Paper, no. 13-027, September 2012, http://nrs.harvard.edu/urn-3:HUL.InstRepos:9547823.

32 Cottingham, Porges, and Richmond, "Shifts in Pelvic Inclination Angle and Parasympathetic Tone."

33 C. M. Meston, and B. B. Gorzalka, "Differential Effects of Sympathetic Activation on Sexual Arousal in Sexually Dysfunctional and Functional Women," *Journal of Abnormal Psychology*, 105, no. 4 (1996), 582–591, doi.org/10.1037/0021-843X.105.4.582.

34 More information on this is available in Ann Diamond Weinstein, *Prenatal Development and Parents' Lived Experiences: How Early Events Shape Our Psychophysiology and Relationships* (New York: W.W. Norton, 2016).

35 Carrière, *Beckenboden, Physiotherapie und Training.* Z. A. Khan, C. Whittal, S. Mansol, Z. A. Lisa Khan, C. Whittal, S. Mansol, L. A. Osborne, P. Reed, and S. Emery, "Effect of Depression and Anxiety on the Success of Pelvic Floor Muscle Training for Pelvic Floor Dysfunction," Journal of Obstetrics and Gynaecology, 33, no. 7 (October 2013), 710–714, doi: 10.3109/01443615.2013.813913. PMID: 24127961.

36 Herbert Benson, *The Relaxation Response* (Neuauflage, NY: William Morrow Paperbacks, 2000).

37   Rudolf Kratzert, *Technik des Klavierspiels: Ein Handbuch Für Pianisten* (Kassel: Bärenreiter Verlag, 2002).

38   Tim Ferris and Derek Sivers, "Tools of Titans: Derek Sivers Distilled," *The Tim Ferris Show*, November 21, 2016, tim. blog/2016/11/21/ tools-of-titans-derek-sivers-distilled/.

39   Volker Stollortz, "Feldenkrais-Methode, Die bewegte Persönlichkeit", Frankfurter Allgemeine, 2 Mai 2014, http://www.faz.net/aktuell/wissen/leben-gene/ feldenkrais-methode-als-bewegungstherapie-12911866.html.

40   Eric Franklin, Bewegung beginnt im Kopf, Seite 17, 3. Auflage, Freiburg: VAK, 2016.

41   Moshé Feldenkrais, *Awareness Through Movement: Easy-to-Do Health Exercises to Improve Your Posture, Vision, Imagination, and Personal Awareness* (New York: Harper & Row, 1977).

42   Lesya Liu, "Neurobites: The 8th Sense," Integrated Listening Systems, December 7, 2017, http://integratedlistening.com/blog/2017/12/07/ neurobites-8th-sense.

43   Katy Bowman, "Butt What About Kegels," Nutritious Movement, May 2020, www.nutritiousmovement.com/1234-we-like-our-pelvic-floor/.

44   Carrière, *Beckenboden, Physiotherapie und Training*.

45   Benita Cantieni, *Tiger Feeling—das sinnliche Beckenbodentraining für sie und ihn* (München: Südwest Verlag, 2003). Isa Herrera, *Female Pelvic Alchemy: Trade Secrets for Energizing Your Love Life, Enhancing Your Pleasure, and Loving Your Body Completely* (New York: Best Seller Publishing, 2017).

46   If you want to explore the jade egg practice I recommend Dr. Saida Désilets, saidadesilets.com

47   Arne Schäffler and Nicole Menche, Mensch—Körper—Krankheit, S. 396. 3. Auflage, München: Urban & Fischer Verlag, 1999.

48   Pschyrembel Medizinisches Wörterbuch, Stichwort »Vagina«, S. 1607, 257. Auflage, Berlin: De Gruyter, 1993.

49   Walther Graumann: CompactLehrbuch Anatomie 3, S. 318, Stuttgart: Schattauer, 2004.

50 The top five of the unloved body parts in Germany: stomach (46%), thighs (30%), buttocks (15%), lower legs (13%) and feet (11%), according to a survey of 1000 Germans, YouGov Deutschland GmbH, "Umfrage: Lediglich 29 Prozent der Männer und 17 Prozent der Frauen fühlen sich wohl in ihrer Haut" Presse Portal, 2008, www.presseportal.de/pm/69450/1310565.

51 Carrière, *Beckenboden, Physiothrapie und Training*.

52 Kristin Linklater, *Freeing the Natural Voice: Imagery and Art in the Practice of Voice and Language* (London: Nick Hern Books, 2006).

53 Caroline Myss, *Chakren, Die Sieben Zentren von Kraft und Heilung* (Munich: Droemer Knaur, 2000).

54 Mantak Chia, *Healing Love through the Tao, Cultivating Female Sexual Energy* (1986; repr. Rochester, NY: Destiny Books, 2005).

55 Michael A. Richard, *Employee Assistance Programs: Wellness/Enhancement Programming*, 4th ed. (New York: Charles C. Thomas Publisher, 2014).

56 Mary Macvean, "'Get Up!' Or Lose Hours of Your Life Every Day, Scientist Says," *Los Angeles Times*, July 31, 2014, http://www.latimes.com/science/sciencenow/la-sci-sn-get-up-20140731-story.html.

57 Dr. James Levine, "Ways Sitting Is Shortening Your Life," *Active Times*, September 5, 2014, www.theactivetimes.com/ways-sitting-shortening-your-life.

58 Ina May Gaskin, *Ina May's Guide to Childbirth: Updated with New Material* (New York: Bantam, 2003)

59 Jonathan Isbit, "Health Benefits of the Natural Squatting Position," *Nature's Platform*, January 2018, www.naturesplatform.com/health_benefits.html.

60 Bernie Clark and Sarah Powers, *The Complete Guide to Yin Yoga: The Philosophy and Practice of Yin Yoga* (Ashland: Wild Strawberry Productions, 2012).

61 Naomi Wolf, *Vagina: A New Biography* (London: Virago, 2012).

62 J. R. Georgiadis, R. Kortekaas, R. Kuipers, A. Nieuwenburg, J. Pruim, A.A. Reinders, and G. Holstege, "Regional Cerebral Blood Flow Changes Associated with Clitorally Induced Orgasm in Healthy Women," *European Journal of Neuroscience*, 24, no. 11 (December 2006), 3305-3316, doi: 10.1111/j.1460-9568.2006.05206.x. PMID: 17156391.

63   Wolf, *Vagina*.

64   Brunhild Hoffmann, *Orgasmus—Die Weibliche Kraft* (München: KOHA Verlag, 2016).

65   University of California Los Angeles, "Key Biobehavioral Pattern Used by Women to Manage Stress," *ScienceDaily*, May 22, 2000, www.sciencedaily.com/ releases/2000/05/000522082151.htm.

66   My description is a synthesis of the current models from Masters and Johnson, Helen Singer Kaplan, Rosemary Basson, and David M. Reed.

67   Andrea Pennington, *The Orgasm Prescription for Women: 21 Days to Heightened Pleasure Deeper Intimacy and Orgasmic Bliss* (Las Vegas: Make Your Mark Global, 2016).

68   Vincent B. van Hasselt and Michel Hersen, *Sourcebook of Psychological Treatment Manuals for Adult Disorders*, S. 348–351 (New York: Springer, 1996).

69   Stefanie Stahl, *Das Kind in dir muss Heimat finden* (München: Kailash, 2015).

70   Herbert Benson, *The Relaxation Response* (New York: William Morrow Paperbacks, 2000). Jayson Gaddis, "The Neuroscience and Power of Safe Relationships—Stephen W. Porges," YouTube, April 19, 2017, youtu.be/3pbVTla932Y.

71   Yuval Noah Harari, *Sapiens: A Brief History of Humankind* (London: Vintage, 2015).

72   Stephen W. Porges: *The Pocket Guide to Polyvagal Theory: The Transformative Power of Feeling Safe* (New York: W.W. Norton, 2017).

73   Alice Miller, Das Drama des Begabten Kindes, Frankfurt: Suhrkamp, 2012 und Die Revolte des Körpers, Frankfurt: Suhrkamp, 2005.

74   Russ Harris, *The Happiness Trap: How to Stop Struggling and Start Living* (Boston: Trumpeter, 2011).

75   Khandis R. Blake, Brock Bastian, Siobhan M. O'Dean, and Thomas F. Denson, "High Estradiol and Low Progesterone Are Associated with High Assertiveness in Women, *Psychoneuroendocrinology*, 75 (2017). S. L. Miller and J. K. Maner, "Scent of a Woman: Men's Testosterone Responses to Olfactory Ovulation Cues," *Psychological Science*, 21, no. 2 (February 2010), 276–283, doi: 10.1177/0956797609357733; epub December 22, 2009, PMID: 20424057.

76   Kerstin Weidner, "Sinkender Hormonspiegel selten für Beschwerden in den Wechseljahren verantwortlich," Uniklinikum Dresden, March 27, 2015, www.uniklinikum-dresden.de/de/presse/aktuelle-medien-informationen/27-marz-2015-sinkender-hormonspiegel-selten-fur-beschwerden-in-den-wechseljahren-verantwortlich.

77   David Rowe and Robert Schulmann, *Einstein on Politics: His Private Thoughts and Public Stands on Nationalism* (Princeton: Princeton University Press, 2007).

78   Wikipedia, "Massage," January 2018, de.wikipedia.org/wiki/Massage.

79   A. Barton, C. Serrao, J. Thompson, et al. "Transabdominal Ultrasound to Assess Pelvic Floor Muscle Performance During Abdominal Curl in Exercising Women," *Int Urogynecol J*, 26 (2015), 1789–1795. doi.org/10.1007/s00192-015-2791-9.

About the author

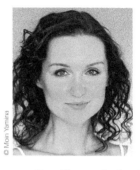

© Moin Yamina

COCO BERLIN is the founder of the Pelvic Floor Integration™ method, the Sensuous Dance Workout™, and Essence of Bellydance™. Her work enables women to connect to their essence and to step into their power.

With her cutting-edge method and fresh approach to women's health and well-being, Coco is a regular guest on German national TV and has worked with brands such as Hilton, L'Oréal, and BMW. Her work has moved over seven million women, and her method is taught by instructors worldwide.

Pussy Yoga is Coco's unique self-study program to help women become more sensual, strong, and confident. *Pussy Yoga* was first published in Germany 2018 and became an instant bestseller, with rave reviews by health professionals and magazines like *Cosmopolitan, Emotion*, and *Jolie*. Coco and her husband have traveled the world for years. Currently, they live in beautiful Valencia, Spain.

FEEL INCREDIBLY
SENSUOUS IN YOUR BODY

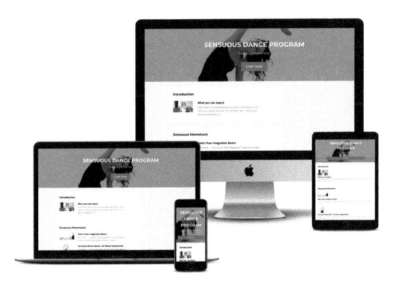

The Sensuous Dance Workout™ by Coco Berlin is your lifestyle program to activate your feminine power and fall in love with yourself.

★ The best practices from Pussy Yoga and many more

★ Video and audio guidance with Coco

★ Online community with Coco

★ Practice anywhere you go

★ Online course for all devices and app for every day

Get it here: Sensuousworkout.com

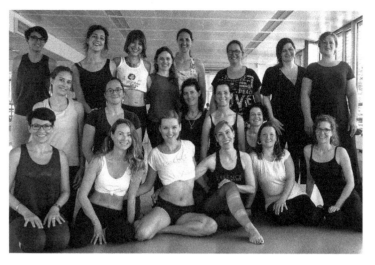

ESSENCE OF BELLYDANCE™ TEACHER TRAINING

Join our growing international community of excellent teachers and coaches.

- ★ Feel amazing in your body and inspire others
- ★ Take your movement technique and your career to the next level
- ★ Become a charismatic performer or teacher
- ★ Step into your power as a leader and as a woman
- ★ Be part of a cutting edge method with international recognition

Essence of Bellydance™ is a new holistic method combining the art of belly dance with Pelvic Floor Integration™, mindfulness and contemporary dance- and bodywork-techniques. Since 2013 we have trained and certified Essence of Bellydance™ teachers from all continents.
And now is your chance!

Join us live or online: Essencebellydance.com